T0192937

Noongar
Bush
Medicine

The Charles and Joy Staples South West Region Publications Fund was established in 1984 on the basis of a generous donation to The University of Western Australia by Charles and Joy Staples.

The purpose of the Fund is to highlight all aspects of the South West region of Western Australia, a geographical area much loved by Charles and Joy Staples, so as to assist the people of the South West region and those in government and private organisations concerned with South West projects to appreciate the needs and possibilities of the region in the widest possible historical perspective.

The fund is administered by a committee whose aims are to make possible the publication by UWA Publishing, of research and writing in any discipline relevant to the South West region.

Charles and Joy Staples South West Region Publications Fund titles

1987
A Tribute to the Group Settlers
Philip E. M. Blond

1992
*For Their Own Good:
Aborigines and government
in the southwest of Western
Australia, 1900-1940*
Anna Haebich

1993
Portraits of the South West
B. K. de Garis

*A Guide to Sources for the
History of South Western
Australia*
compiled by Ronald Richards

1994
*Jardee: The Mill That Cheated
Time* Doreen Owens

1995
*Dearest Isabella: Life and
Letters of Isabella Ferguson,
1819-1910*
Prue Joske

*Blacklegs: The Scottish Colliery
Strike of 1911*
Bill Latter

1997
*Barefoot in the Creek: A Group
Settlement Childhood in
Margaret River*
L. C. Burton

*Ritualist on a Tricycle:
Frederick Goldsmith, Church,
Nationalism and Society in
Western Australia* Colin Holden

*Western Australia as it is Today,
1906.* Leopoldo Zunini, Royal
Consul of Italy edited and
translated by Richard Bosworth
and Margot Melia

2002
*The South West from Dawn till
Dusk* Rob Olver

2003
*Contested Country: a history
of the Northcliffe area, Western
Australia* Patricia Crawford and
Ian Crawford

2004
*Orchard and Mill: The Story of
Bill Lee, South-West Pioneer*
Lyn Adams

2005
*Richard Spencer: Napoleonic
War Naval Hero and Australian
Pioneer* Gwen Chessell

2006
A Story to Tell
Laurel Nannup (reprinted 2012)

2008
*Alexander Collie: Colonial
Surgeon, Naturalist and
Explorer*
Gwen Chessell

*The Zealous Conservator: A
Life of Charles Lane Poole*
John Dargavel

2009
*It's Still in our Heart This is Our
Country: The Single Noongar
Claim History*
John Host and Chris Owen

*Shaking Hands on the Fringe:
Negotiating the Aboriginal
World at King George's Sound*
Tiffany Shellam

2011
Noongar Mambara Bakitj
Kim Scott and Wirlomin
Noongar Language and
Stories Project

Mamang
Kim Scott and Wirlomin
Noongar Language and
Stories Project

Guy Grey-Smith: Life Force
Andrew Gaynor

2013
Dwoort Baal Kaat
Kim Scott and Wirlomin
Noongar Language and Stories
Project

Yira Boornak Nyininy
Kim Scott and Wirlomin
Noongar Language and Stories
Project

2014
*A Boy's Short Life: The Story Of
Warren Braedon/Louis Johnson*
Anna Haebich and Steve Mickler

*Plant Life on the Sandplains: A
Global Biodiversity Hotspot*
Hans Lambers

*Fire and Hearth (revised
facsimile edition)* Sylvia Hallam

The Lake's Apprentice
Annamaria Weldon

2015
*Running Out: Water in Western
Australia* Ruth Morgan

*A Journey Travelled:
Aboriginal-European Relations
At Albany And Surrounding
Regions From First Colonial
Contact To 1926*
Murray Arnold

*The Southwest: Australia's
Biodiversity Hotspot*
Victoria Laurie

*Invisible Country: South-West
Australia: Understanding a
Landscape* Bill Bunbury

Noongar Bush Medicine

MEDICINAL PLANTS OF THE SOUTH-WEST OF WESTERN AUSTRALIA

VIVIENNE HANSEN AND
JOHN HORSFALL

First published in 2016 by
UWA Publishing
Crawley, Western Australia 6009
www.uwap.uwa.edu.au
UWAP is an imprint of UWA Publishing
a division of The University of Western Australia

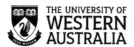

National Library of Australia Cataloguing-in-Publication entry
Creator: Hansen, Vivienne, author.
Title: Noongar bush medicine plants : medicinal plants of the south-
west of Western Australia / Vivienne Hansen, John Horsfall.

ISBN: 9781742589060 (paperback)

Subjects: Medicinal plants--Western Australia--South-West. Plants,
Useful--Western Australia--South-West. Materia medica, Vegetable-
-Western Australia--South-West. Noongar (Australian people)--
Medicine--Western Australia--South-West.

Other Creators/Contributors: Horsfall, John, 1945- author.

Printed by McPhersons Printing Group
Design by Upside Creative
Front cover photo: Starflower, *Calytrix strigose*,
                     photographer Ivan Holliday

Back cover photos: Mottlecah, *Eucalyptus macrocarpa*,
                     photographer Tatiana Gerus

                     Guinea Flower, *Hibbertia glomerosa*,
                     photographer John Tann

                     Slender banksia, *Banksia attenuate*,
                     photographer Ivan Holliday

Page 26 photo: Bloodroot, *Haemodorum spicatum* R.Br.,
                     photographer Sian Mawson

Contents

Disclaimer

This book has been written based on information accumulated by the authors from personal knowledge passed on from family members; third parties, including websites, records and documents that other parties have prepared; and Indigenous elders with traditional healing knowledge. While the authors have made their best endeavours to produce an accurate account of plants used medicinally by the Indigenous people of the south-west of Western Australia, they do not warrant or make any claim as to the accuracy or otherwise of the information contained in the work and accept no responsibility whatsoever for any inaccurate information contained in the book. It is the authors' recommendation that people wishing to collect or cultivate the plants described in this book and use them for medicinal purposes for themselves, their family or their friends should consult with elders and traditional healers who have knowledge of the plants in their area before doing so.

Preface

Vivienne 'Binyarn' Hansen (née Bennell) was born in Beverley, Western Australia, into a traditional, large Noongar family, including Bennells and McGuires, Collards, Haydens, Reidys and other Noongar families in and around Brookton and other country towns to which the families had relocated. She and I had a strong link to Noongar heritage and culture through our great-grandfathers, grandfathers, great-grandmothers, grandmothers, parents, uncles and aunties, who were fiercely dedicated to retaining our spiritual and natural Noongar ways.

Binyarn's early days were spent around the Brookton reserves and Peppers farm, out near Aldersyde, where we would spend hours experimenting with anything that we thought was interesting, except the rotten duck eggs that would explode and we would smell of "Goona" (faeces). The good bush camps of mia-mias and humpies were built in amongst the Mangart (Jam Wattle) trees, the Teatree bushes, and the Sheoak trees. To this day we are very proud of our success, brought about through our strong upbringing in and around the bush camps.

Our elders were strong willed about our upbringing, on the grounds of discipline and strong family morals. Binyarn and her brother Greg were raised by Pop Clarrie and Nanna Olive McGuire in Brookton, and as it is with strong family association, we assisted and supported each other. Binyarn was a strong-willed girl, who grew into a strong-willed woman, who became heavily involved in Noongar culture and heritage that our families shared with us during our upbringing. This clearly shows in the development of this book, her learning and understanding of bush tucker and bush medicine and her producing outstanding items within her learning.

This learning was taken from the early days, in the 1950s, as our Noongar families travelled around the bush – working, clearing land and shearing in the farms around Brookton, west Brookton, Aldersyde, Kweda (itself the Noongar name of a plant) and other places; camping in the bush; being taught the old, wise ways of our elders; being told, 'You can't eat that', 'This is medicine', 'This is good tucker', in relation to environmental plants; learning the art of which animals supplied the best oils and medicines that could be used for sore muscles, headaches and tummy aches; what gums to use for constipation, what gums to use to stop belly aches; when to use Sandalwood and Quandong seeds; and many other useful recipes that were passed on from our large Noongar families. During this time Binyarn met and married her husband, Mort Hansen, and raised her family of children, who now have children of their own and in whose upbringing Binyarn still plays an active part.

Today Binyarn spends much of her time developing her bush medicines and passing on her knowledge to the community, which is so important in this day and age – not keeping the secrets but passing it on to other members of the family to learn and to assist in the production of her medicines and ointments.

Binyarn is a very proud Noongar with strong cultural and heritage values which she has shared. I am a very proud relation and proud to call Binyarn my sister, and Mort brother.

A very special thank you to John for his dedication and support towards my sister, and I congratulate them both for their work.

Neville Collard

About the Authors

Vivienne's Story

I am a Balladong Wadjuk Yorga from the Bibbulmun Nation, or Noongar people, of the south-west of Western Australia. I was born in Beverley, and my childhood was spent in Brookton and the surrounding regions of Noongar country. My mother was Myrtle, who was the youngest child of Kate Collard and Norman Bennell, and it was they who raised me until my grandmother died. After the death of my grandmother, I went to live with my mother's sister, Aunty Olive, and her husband, Uncle Clarrie McGuire. These family members and older uncles, aunts and cousins raised me to have a strong sense of respect, appreciation and knowledge of Noongar identity, culture and language. Like all my relatives, this close connection to country enabled me to explore the local bushlands and develop a deep understanding and knowledge of traditional bush medicine, remedies and practices.

Grandfather was a healer, like his father before him, and he and his two brothers, Granny Felix and Granny Bert told us stories about our Noongar people and culture. They taught us how to look for signs in our surrounds, such as the abundance of the blossoms on the gum trees, which could tell us about the coming seasons and weather patterns. My grandfather Norman and his brothers taught us about other signs and how to hunt for possum and goanna. We were also taught how to perform certain cultural ceremonies when we are near water or places of special significance. This was to acknowledge the land, our Mother Earth, for all she provides for our people.

My aunties and older cousins took us walking through the bush, where we gathered the berries and yams, collected gum and sucked the sweet nectar from the flowers of certain

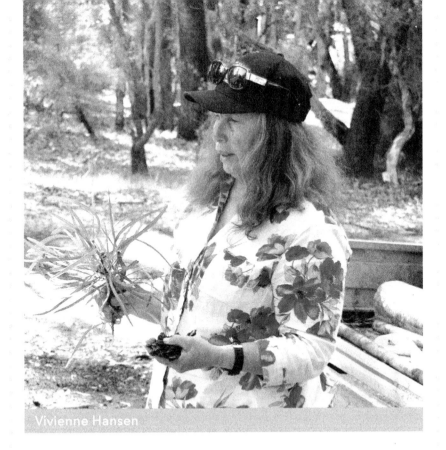

Vivienne Hansen

trees and plants when they were in season. Even today, the seasons play a vital role in medicine, as some plants are only available after a rainy season or need fire to regrow. We were taught to just collect what we need at that particular time; there is no need to cut an entire tree down when we simply require a handful of leaves. I also learnt that it was very important not to trespass on another group's area without their permission.

After Nanna Kate's death, life with my aunt and uncle continued along these same ways, but we got to go out in the bush more regularly, as Uncle Clarrie worked on a lot of farms around Brookton. At this time in my life, many of the farms had an abundance of bushland, as much of the land had not been cleared for crops. One of the farms we lived on was right next door to the state forest between Brookton and Kelmscott. Our time there gave me many opportunities to explore the bush and the plants that grew there, and I was always asking Uncle and Aunt what they were used for. I did not always get answers to all my questions, but that is when my interest in native plants began to grow and the foundations were laid for my work in this area today.

In 2008, I undertook formal training at the Marr Mooditj Foundation and completed Certificate IV in Bush and Western Herbal Medicine. I am very proud to have been the first Indigenous member of the National Herbalist Association of Australia and a presenter at the 7th International Conference on Herbal Medicine 2012, in Coolangatta, Queensland.

While enrolled at Marr Mooditj, I became aware that much of the information published on Aboriginal bush medicine did not contain a great deal of information on Noongar medicines and that the majority of the works published were by non-Aboriginal authors. This ignited a desire within me to gather and compile information on plants that our ancestors used in Noongar country. My desire was to produce a document using information gathered from published records and from my own empirical knowledge, which can be used as a reference and, even more importantly, as a historical record for all our Noongar people.

I believe that this compilation, which I have created with the assistance of John, is a unique body of work. We have only covered the bare minimum of plants in Noongar country, but we would love to see this work encourage other Noongar people to do the same and in so doing broaden the knowledge about our beautiful culture and country, so that it won't be lost.

Sharing cultural knowledge is an important aspect of my life, and I really enjoy having opportunities to pass the knowledge on to my family and the wider community. I also draw a great deal of pleasure from seeing how my work benefits others, especially in improving their health and wellbeing.

Nowadays, I am often accompanied by family members, especially my young grandchildren and great-grandchildren, when I return to the places where I grew up. I share my stories with them, thereby ensuring that my knowledge is passed down to the next generation.

I attribute my passion and knowledge of bush medicine to my grandparents and family elders and to the ongoing support of my husband, Morton, and family. All of my knowledge is based on my interpretation of Noongar botanical practices handed down to me by my ancestors.

John's Story

My first contact with an Australian Indigenous community was in 1963, when I spent two years with the Warnindilyakwa people, who speak the Anindilyakwa language, on Groote Eylandt, in the Northern Territory. I was employed by BHP and later Groote Eylandt Mining Company but spent many hours during my days off hunting and fishing with the men of the island. While on the island, I couldn't help noticing how fit and healthy the Warnindilyakwa people were. Although the people lived at the Anglican missions at Angurugu and Umbakumba, they often spent long periods away from the missions, hunting, fishing, crabbing and gathering bush tucker, and getting plenty of exercise doing so. They also had good access to bush medicines.

Not long after commencing my nursing training in 1967, I became interested in alternative medicine and completed a diploma in Naturopathy and Herbal Medicine. While researching for session notes for one of the subjects I was teaching for the bachelor's degree in Indigenous Community

xiv

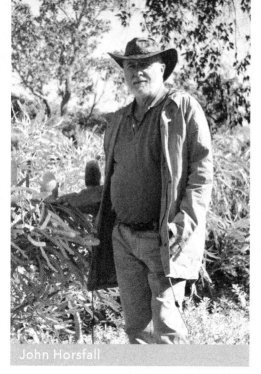

John Horsfall

Health at Curtin University titled 'Bush Medicine', I noticed that, although there were books covering Australian medicinal herbs and some covering Western Australian medicinal herbs, there was very little coverage of medicinal plants used by the Noongar people of south-west Western Australia. This book is intended to fill that gap by presenting an inventory of medicinal herbs that were used by the Noongar people of the Bibbulmun Nation.

The authors wish to acknowledge the help of a multitude of people, Indigenous and non-Indigenous, without whose help it would have been impossible to write this book.

Vivienne would like to thank the following people for the tremendous support, advice and encouragement they gave her while she was working on this book: her husband, Morton Hansen, her children and grandchildren, and Uncle Theo Michael, Neville Collard, Winnie McHenry, Janet Hayden, Carol Garlett and Sandra Kremple.

John would like to thank his wife, Kamala Horsfall, and family for their encouragement and support while he was writing this book.

William Archer, who manages the Esperance Wildflowers blog, assisted with descriptions of the plants found around Esperance. His assistance is greatly appreciated. For those interested in wildflowers of the south-west, the blog can be found at www.esperancewildflowers.blogspot.com.au. It contains many photographs and descriptions of the beautiful wildflowers that grow in the Esperance area.

Malcolm French, the author of *Eucalypts of Western Australia's Wheatbelt,* assisted greatly by supplying beautiful photographs of some of the eucalypts. His book and annual *EucMedia* newsletters, about Western Australian eucalypts, can be obtained through his website: www.eucalyptsofwa.com.au.

Thanks also to all those photographers who gave permission to use their beautiful photographs for the illustrations, including Russell Dahms, William Archer, Andrew Hodgson, Russell Cummings, Bill and Mark Bell, Alfred Sin, Friends of Chiltern Mt Pilot National Park, Tatiana Gerus, Alison Doley, Jean Hort, Leif Stridvall and numerous others.

xvi

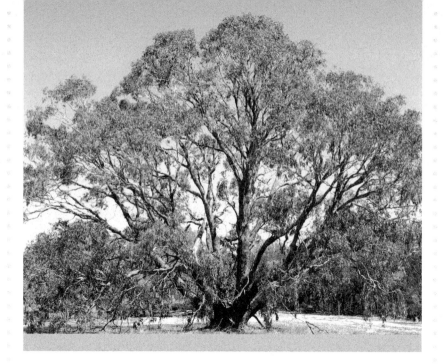

A special thanks to the Noongar Boodjar Language Cultural Aboriginal Corporation, at the Batchelor Institute of Indigenous Tertiary Education, for allowing us to use their map of the Noongar dialect regions. Their website can be found at noongarboodjar.com.au.

Vivienne proudly acknowledges her Noongar heritage and wishes to pay her respects to her people past and present and declares this land she dwells on is and always will be the land of the Bibbulman Nation.

The country of the Noongar people, Aboriginal Australians of the south-west of Western Australia, stretches from Geraldton to Esperance, comprising an area of land of approximately 3 million hectares, with a coastline that covers 16,000 kilometres. According to Noongar elders, the islands of Carnac, Garden and Rottnest were created when the oceans swept in and separated them from the mainland. Traditionally, Noongar people had their own language, laws and customs and gathered regularly for celebrations, trade, marriage arrangements and other purposes. They lived well in their country, with a varied diet depending on the season and location.

For over 50,000 years before colonisation, the Noongar people were much healthier than most Aboriginal Australians are today. Living in the open, in a land largely free from disease, they benefited from a better diet, more exercise, less stress and a supportive community. With colonisation came many diseases, such as measles, mumps, diphtheria and whooping cough, and sexually transmitted infections, all of which reached epidemic proportions in some communities. Aboriginal Australians were very susceptible to respiratory diseases, and after colonisation, flu and tuberculosis caused many deaths and contributed immensely to the decline of the Aboriginal population, as there were no developed medicines to treat them. Traditional herbal medicine was of course ineffective against these introduced diseases (Cribb & Cribb, 1983).

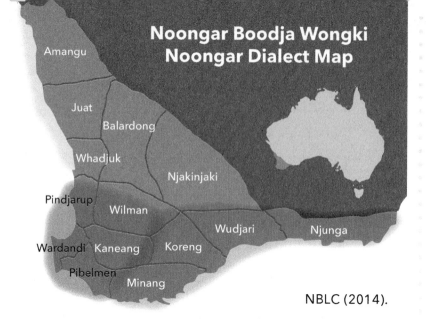

Noongar Boodja Wongki
Noongar Dialect Map

Amangu

Juat

Balardong

Whadjuk

Njakinjaki

Pindjarup

Wilman

Wudjari

Njunga

Wardandi Kaneang Koreng

Pibelmen

Minang

NBLC (2014).

Dialect groups

According to Tindale (1940), Noongar country is occupied by fourteen different dialect groups (see the map above), which he identified as Amangu, Ballardong (Balardong on the map), Yued, Kaneang, Koreng, Mineng, Njakinjaki, Njunga, Pibelmen, Binjareb, Wardandi, Whadjuk (Minang on map), Wilman and Wudjari. The Noongar (Pindjarup on map) people traditionally spoke dialects of the Noongar language, a member of the large Pama-Nyungan language family. The Pama-Nyungan languages are the most widespread family of Indigenous Australian languages, containing perhaps 300 languages. The name 'Pama-Nyungan' is derived from the names of the two most widely separated groups: the Pama languages of the north-east and the Nyungan languages of the south-west. The words *pama* and *nyunga* 'man' in their respective languages (Frawley, 2004).

The spelling Noongar was supported by Great Southern people at a meeting in Narrogin in 1992 and remains in common use on the south coast and Great Southern regions of Western Australia. Other spellings that have been used include Nyungar, Nyoongar, Nyoongah, Nyungah, Nyugah, Yungar and Noonga (NBLC, 2014).

Seasons

There are six seasons for Noongar people, and their calendar, outlined below, is extremely important to all Noongar people, as it is a guide to what nature is doing at every stage of the year, as well as an aid in respecting the land in relation to plant and animal fertility cycles and land and animal preservation. For example, Noongar law required that no seed-bearing plants be dug up until after flowering. The Noongar people knew when the seasons changed by the weather patterns, the movement of the stars, the behaviour of the birds and the lifecycle of the plants.

The Noongar Seasons

Season	Months	Weather	Activities
Birak	December, January	Hot and dry	Sections of scrubland were burnt to force animals into the open.
Bunuru	February, March	Hottest part of the year, with warm easterly winds and sparse rainfall throughout.	Families moved to estuaries for fishing.
Djeran	April, May	Cooler, pleasant weather begins.	People continued fishing, and collected bulbs and seeds for food.

Season	Months	Weather	Activities
Makuru	June, July	Cold fronts continue. Usually the wettest part of the year. The rains replenish inland water resources.	Kangaroos and emus were hunted for their red meat and skins that were used for warm clothing.
Djilba	August, September	Usually the coldest part of the year, with clear, cold days and nights and warmer, rainy and windy periods.	People collected roots, and hunted emus, possums and kangaroos.
Kambarang	October, November	Longer dry periods, with fewer cold fronts crossing the coast.	People moved towards the coast and caught frogs, tortoises and freshwater crayfish.

Adapted from Rainbow Coast (2015).

Animal and plant use

Noongar people enjoyed a diverse diet, which was based on the seasons. Kangaroos, ducks and fish were abundant, as were turtles, marron, emus, turkeys, wallabies, snakes and lizards. Fish traps were used to catch fish, and firestick farming was practised to improve the grass and drive out small game. Noongar people had an intimate knowledge of edible plants and when and where they could be found. Some of the plants were potentially poisonous, but Noongar people knew what to do in order to make them edible. Wattle, Eucalypt, Banksia, Grevillea and Melaleuca trees provided nectar that was taken from the flowers either by sucking them directly or by soaking them in water to make a sweet drink called *neip*.

Trees also provided the materials necessary for the making of implements, such as spears, boomerangs, digging sticks and bowls. Bark shelters were built in cold winters, and bark was used to wrap food for cooking. The Noongar people carried firesticks when travelling long distances from the camps (*kullarks*). They were used to start fires to keep warm in the cold. When it rained, the firesticks were usually carried under cloaks. Gum from Grass Trees was used in making stone implements for a variety of purposes. The stone was quarried from a wide area. Grinding stones, spears, quartz rocks, ochres and clays were very popular trading items for Noongar people.

The Noongar people wore kangaroo-skin cloaks (*booka*) for warmth. The skins were pegged out on the ground to dry then cut with a stone knife into the desired shapes and the inner surfaces scraped until the skins became very soft and pliable. Once this was completed, the skins were sewn together with animal sinews and rubbed with grease and red ochre.

Knowledge of the medicinal uses of plants has kept Noongar people in good health for thousands of years. Knowing what to use to treat particular ailments extends beyond the plant kingdom and includes other types of food, animal oils, healing rituals such as smoking ceremonies, and healers. Noongars were mainly hunters and gatherers, dependent on the environment for food supply, moving from place to place within defined boundaries. Tribal boundaries were not crossed, and the seasons played a vital role in medicine, as some plants were available only after a rainy season or needed fire for regrowth. Noongar people carried no medicine kits and had to have readily available remedies that could be used when needed. They were able to heal with whatever plants were in the locality of their camp. Their knowledge and skills of the plants, environment, seasons and animals around them were parts of their everyday life skills needed to survive.

Physical, spiritual, social and emotional wellbeing

The Noongar people used many substances to enhance their wellbeing, including fire (*kaarl*); smoking (*booyi or kir*); charcoal (*kop* or *yaarkal*); ash (*yoort*) and coals (*birdal*); ochres and clay (*darduk*); mud, sand and termite dirt; animal fats and oils; and plants.

Fire played an integral role in the lives of Noongar people. It was used medicinally, spiritually and cosmetically. It provided light in the darkness of night and warmth on cold evenings and was the central focus for the passing on of knowledge from generation to generation, which was done sitting around campfires. Fires burning at night also provided protection from mosquitoes and other insects and were used to keep bad spirits away from the camp. It has played an important role in the healing process of the Noongar people.

Ceremonies using smoke were performed on newborn babies to keep them safe and make them grow up strong and healthy; babies were also rubbed with oils to render them stronger. Often, nursing mothers were smoked or steamed (HLPG, 2010) to strengthen their bodies during that

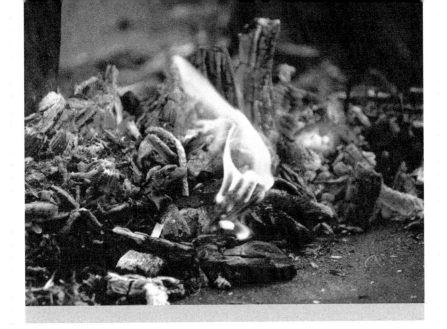

period in their lives. Leaves, twigs and small branches were heated over hot coals to release their oils, and the vapours were then inhaled.

Ashes, steam pits and steam beds were used medicinally. A steam pit was made by digging out a shallow pit, making a fire and then removing the ashes from the fire, lining the pit with leaves and placing kangaroo skins over the top. The sick person lay on top of the skins and was then covered with a further kangaroo skin.

Ochres were used mainly in ceremonies but sometimes in bush medicine. White ochre (*yoort* or *dardark*) was used for decoration of the body for ceremonial dance purposes. Certain soils were used medicinally, and some were also applied to the skin for protection from sunburn.

Emu (*weitj*) and goanna (*karda*) fat was an essential ingredient in many medicinal remedies and was considered to be a powerful healing agent for all health problems. It was applied directly to areas of pain and to wounds. Animal fat was also used to soften the skin.

There was great richness and diversity in the vegetation within Noongar country, and the Noongar people were able to

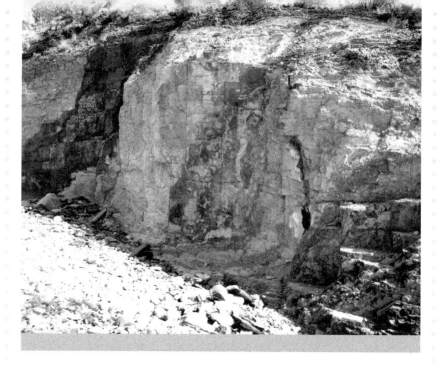

extract various saps and liquids from the plants and the earth to treat sickness. The methods of extraction and usage varied as the environments and seasons changed. Leafy branches were often placed over a fire while the patient squatted on top and inhaled the steam. Sprigs of aromatic leaves might be crushed and the smell inhaled, or the leaves would be inserted into the nose or placed into a pillow on which the patient slept. To make an infusion, leaves, flowers, twigs or bark were crushed and soaked in water which was then drunk or washed over the body. Ointment was prepared by mixing crushed leaves with animal fat. Other treatments included rubbing down the patient with crushed seed paste, fruit pulp or animal oil, or dripping milky sap or a gummy solution over them. Most plant medicines were externally applied (Cribb & Cribb, 1983). Except in ointments, medicines were rarely mixed. Very occasionally, two plants were used together. Noongar medicines were never measured, and there were no specific times of treatment; as most remedies were also applied externally, there was little risk of overdosing or poisoning.

Healing practices

Noongar people often had need of bush medicines. Sleeping at night by fires meant they sometimes suffered from burns. Strong sunshine and certain foods caused headaches, and eye infections were common. Feasting on sour fruits or rancid meat brought on digestive upsets, and although tooth decay was not a big problem, coarse, gritty food may have worn teeth down. The Noongar people were also occasionally stung by jellyfish, insects and other creatures, and bitten by snakes. In the bush, there was always a chance of injury, and fighting sometimes may have ended in bruises, gashes and open wounds (Cribb & Cribb, 1983).

The healing of trivial, non-spiritual complaints and minor illnesses using herbs and other remedies was practised by all Aboriginal Australians, although older women were usually the experts. To ensure success, plants were often prescribed side by side with magic (Cribb & Cribb, 1983). One of the main features of traditional Noongar society was the role of the doctors, who had the power of healing through their hands, and the Noongar people believed that they also had the power to drive away rain or wind, bring down lightning or cause harm to an individual. Traditional healers sometimes employed herbs in their rites.

To deal with ailments, Noongar people used a range of remedies, which included medicinal plants, steam baths, clay pits, charcoal and mud, massages and secret chants (Cribb & Cribb, 1983). Many of the remedies did directly heal. Aromatic herbs, tannin-rich inner barks and resins, or gums (kinos) have well-documented therapeutic effects. Other plants undoubtedly harboured alkaloids or other compounds with pronounced healing effects. Unfortunately, very few native remedies have been tested systematically (Lassak &

McCarthy, 2001). Below is a list of traditional remedies used for various complaints:

Aching joints were relieved with heated plant poultices, hot mud, or red ochre (*wilgi* or *mirda*) mixed with animal fat. Goanna fat was highly prized for the healing of painful joints.

Ailing health was treated by eating cooked bobtail (*yoorn*), goanna and echidna (*nyingarn*).

Backaches were relieved using gum poultices.

Broken limbs were set in a jacket of mud and clay then bound tightly between sheets of bark.

Burns were treated by smearing sap from certain plants, animal fat, saliva or mud on the affected parts.

Coughs and colds were relieved by inhaling the vapours from the crushed leaves of specific plants, especially Eucalypts. Steam pits and steam beds were also used for the treatment of colds.

Diarrhoea and constipation were relieved by consuming small amounts of gum from a Eucalypt.

Earaches were relieved by pouring decoctions of certain plant parts into the ear canal.

Eye pain was treated with breast milk or with the crushed leaves of certain plants moistened with water or saliva.

Fevers were relieved by bathing the sufferer with infusions of crushed leaves.

Headaches could be cured by inhaling vapours from the crushed leaves of some plants, by rubbing the crushed leaves on the head, by drinking decoctions of certain plants, by sleeping in the smoke from a fire, or by externally applying red ochre mixed with animal fat.

Heartburn was relieved by chewing and swallowing charcoal; this also aided digestion.

Muscle aches were treated with heated stones placed upon them. This remedy was also used for other sore parts of the body.

Poisons that had been ingested were countered by chewing and swallowing charcoal.

Rashes were relieved with heated plant poultices, hot mud, or the fat from the echidna and possum (*koomoorl*, *goormoorl* or *goomal*) rubbed on the skin.

Rheumatic problems were alleviated by lying on a bed of green leaves. Steam pits and steam beds were also used for the treatment of rheumatism.

Skin problems were treated with external application of red ochre mixed with animal fat.

Snake bites were countered with directly applied ash.

Stings and bites were treated by applying gum leaves that had been heated over fire.

Toothache was relieved by using a mouthwash or by chewing the leaves of certain plants. Charcoal was chewed to clean the teeth.

Wounds in the forms of ordinary cuts and grazes were treated by poultices of crushed leaves, mud, clay or ash. Crushed gum from Eucalypts would also be sprinkled on wounds to stem bleeding, and wounds were disinfected or cauterised with a burning stick. Specific types of soils were applied directly to open wounds or as poultices to retard infection. Wounds were also sometimes dressed with ochre or clay.

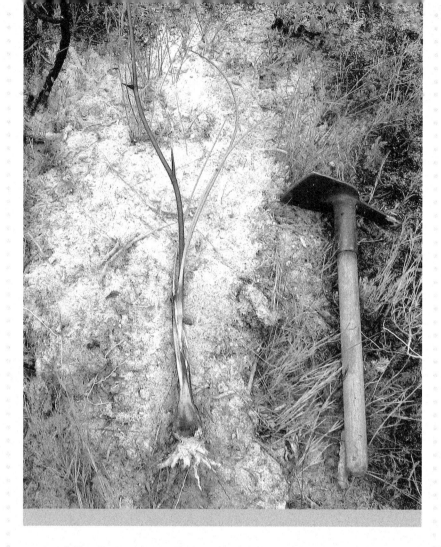

In the following pages, the authors have recorded information on many of the medicinal plants that were regularly used by the Noongar people of the south-west of Western Australia. They hope it will ensure that the traditional knowledge is not lost forever with the passing of elders and traditional healers.

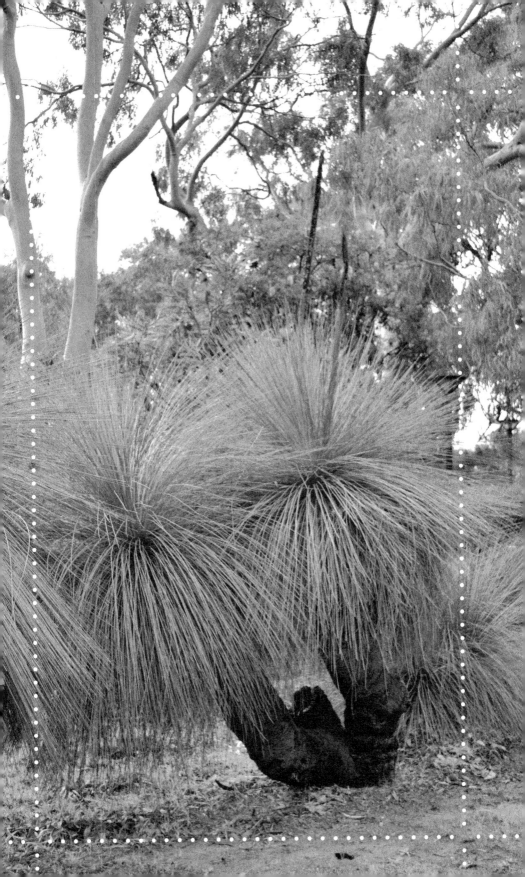

Acorn Banksia

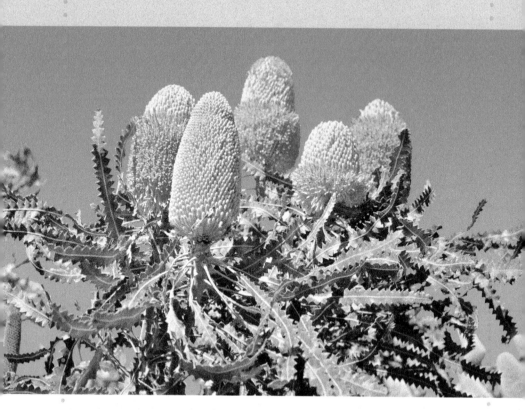

Botanical Name *Banksia prionotes* Lindl.

Common Name Acorn Banksia.

Noongar Name Manyret.

Description Acorn Banksia grows as a tree or shrub up to 10 m high. The leaves are about 150–300 mm long and 20 mm wide. The flower spikes are cylindrical and very conspicuous. The flowers have a distinct acorn shape (hence the name) and when fully open are an orange colour and about 100–150 mm long and 80 mm in diameter. The flowers usually appear during autumn and winter (late Bunuru to early Djilba). This species is fire sensitive and cannot regenerate if it is burnt in a bushfire, so it relies on seed to regenerate (ANPSA, 2016).

Family Proteaceae Juss.

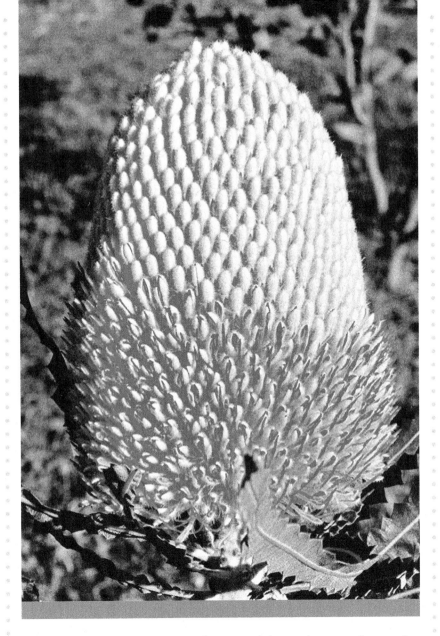

Habitat Acorn Banksia prefers sand, loam, brown clay and laterite over granite. It inhabits sandplains, sand dunes and undulating slopes (FloraBase, 2016).

Distribution Acorn Banksia is native to the south-west of Western Australia and is found from Shark Bay to the Wongan Hills (ANPSA, 2016).

Uses For the Noongar people's use of Banksias, see page 16.

Banksias

The Banksias are named after Sir Joseph Banks (1743-1820), a prominent naturalist and botanist who was on the *Endeavour* with Captain James Cook on his voyage to the east coast of Australia in 1770. All Banksias but one are found only in Australia. Sixty of the Australian Banksias are native only to the south-west of Western Australia. The eastern and western Banksias are quite separate species (ANBG & CANBR, 2012). The Banksias listed in this book were all used in similar ways by the Noongar people, as described below.

Parts Used
The flowers.

Medicinal Uses
Infusions of the flowers (made by steeping them in water) were drunk to relieve coughs and sore throats (City of Joondalup, 2011).

Other Uses
Infusions of the flower spikes made sweet, refreshing drinks (City of Joondalup, 2011).

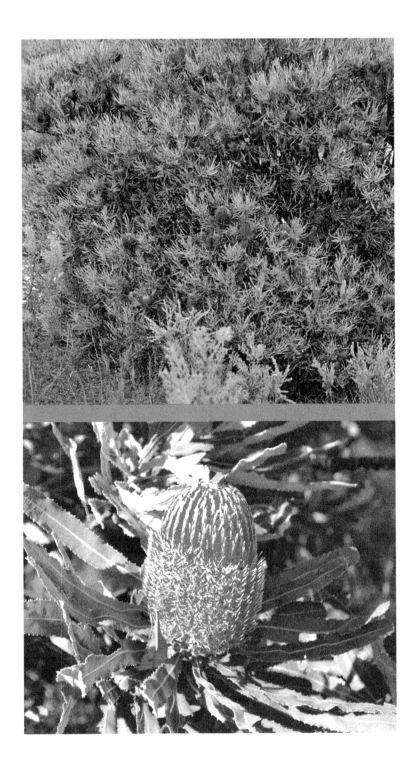

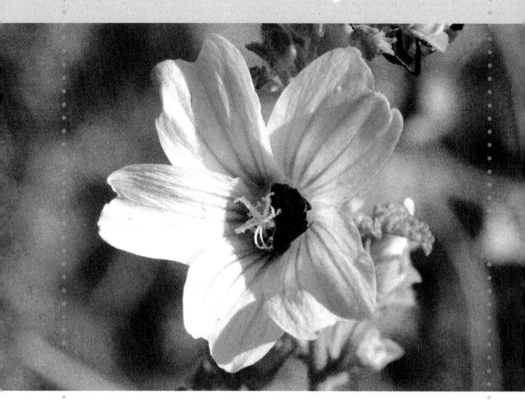

Family Malvaceae Juss.

Botanical Names *Malva preissiana* Miq., formerly *Lavatera plebeia.*

Common Names Australian Hollyhock and Native Marshmallow.

Noongar Names Not known for this plant.

Description Australian Hollyhock is a sturdy, erect, open shrub that grows to around 2 m tall. It is annual or biennial, meaning it takes one or two years to complete its biological cycle. The leaves are oval or kidney shaped and around 60 mm long; they feel soft and downy. The flowers are about 50 mm across and white in the Perth region; when found inland they may be mauve. The fruits are disc-like and segmented, with up to fifteen segments, each containing one seed (Rippey & Rowland, 1995).

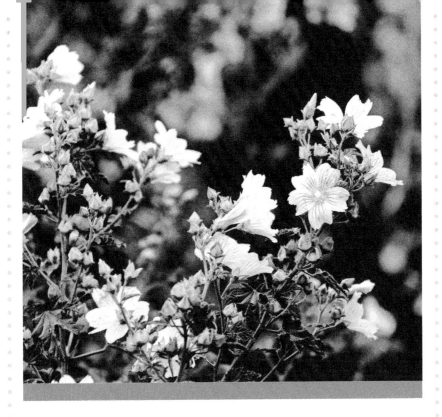

Habitat Australian Hollyhock grows in a variety of soils, including sand, clay and loam over granite and limestone. It is found in various habitats that include islands, plains and valleys. (FloraBase, 2016).

Distribution Australian Hollyhock is found on the south-west coastal strip and on islands from Dirk Hartog Island to Busselton. An inland variant can be found from Coolgardie through South Australia, Victoria, New South Wales and southern Queensland (Rippey & Rowland, 1995).

Parts Used The flowers, leaves and roots.

Medicinal Uses The fresh flowers were eaten or infusions of the flowers taken internally to reduce digestive, respiratory and urinary tract inflammation (Rippey & Rowland, 1995). Poultices of the boiled leaves were used to treat sores and boils (Lassak & McCarthy, 2001).

Other Uses The roots were eaten as food by Aboriginals in South Australia (Rippey & Rowland, 1995).

Botanical Name *Spinifex longifolius* R.Br.

Common Names Beach Spinifex and Long Leaved Spinifex.

Noongar Names Not known for this plant.

Other Aboriginal Names Wurruwarduwarda (Lassak & McCarthy, 2001).

Description Beach Spinifex is a coarse grass with long, thin leaves that grow up to 300 mm in length. There are male and female plants. The rhizomatous roots spread through the sand, forming the grass into large tussocks (Rippey & Rowland, 1995). The green-brown flower spikes, barely 10 mm long, appear from April to January (Djeran to Birak) (FloraBase, 2016).

Habitat Beach Spinifex prefers white sand on coastal sand dunes (FloraBase, 2016).

Distribution Beach Spinifex is found along the northern coast from Northern Queensland and the Northern Territory down along the west coast to Perth. It is also found on Rottnest, Garden, Carnac, Seal and Penguin islands and in New Guinea and Indonesia (Rippey & Rowland, 1995).

Parts Used The leaves and young tips, or shoots.

Medicinal Uses Juice from the young tips, obtained by squeezing them with the fingers, was allowed to drip into the eyes to relieve soreness from conjunctivitis. Infusions of the crushed leaves were also used to bathe sore eyes (Lassak & McCarthy, 2001).

Family Poaceae Barnhart & Barnh.

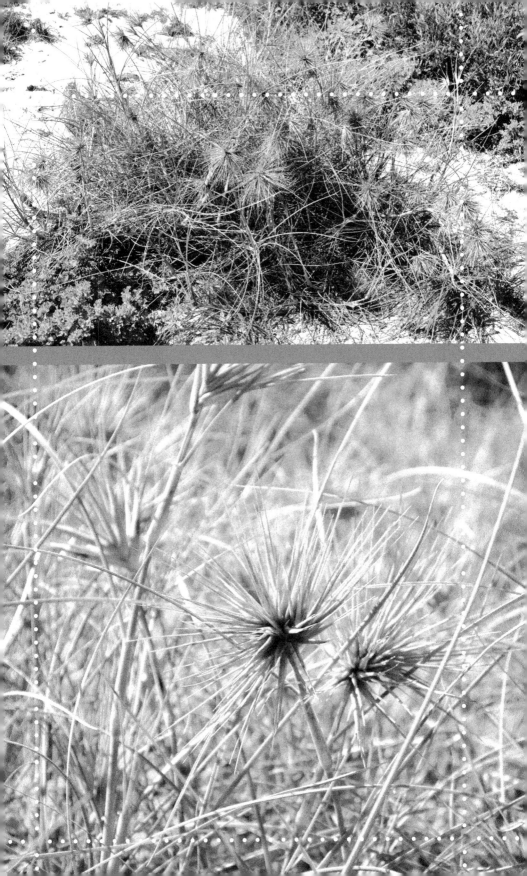

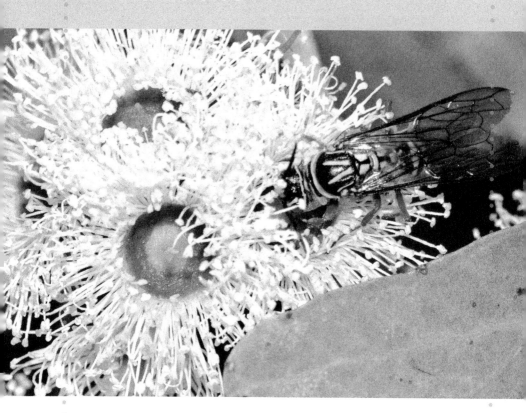

Family **Myrtaceae Juss.**

Botanical Name *Eucalyptus todtiana* F.Muell.

Common Names Blackbutt, Coastal Blackbutt and Pricklybark (Bennett, 1991).

Noongar Names Dwutta, Maynee (Cunningham, 2005) and Morl (Bindon & Chadwick, 2011).

Description Blackbutt grows to about 15 m tall, either as a tree (single trunk) or as a mallee (multiple trunks). It has rough, fibrous, greyish brown bark with longitudinal furrows. Its greyish green leaves are long and lance shaped. It produces cream and white, spiky flowers from January to April (late Birak to early Djeran). The fruits are globular, mottled green gumnuts (FloraBase, 2016).

Habitat Blackbutt generally occurs near the crests of low, sandy rises in white, grey and yellow sand and laterite in

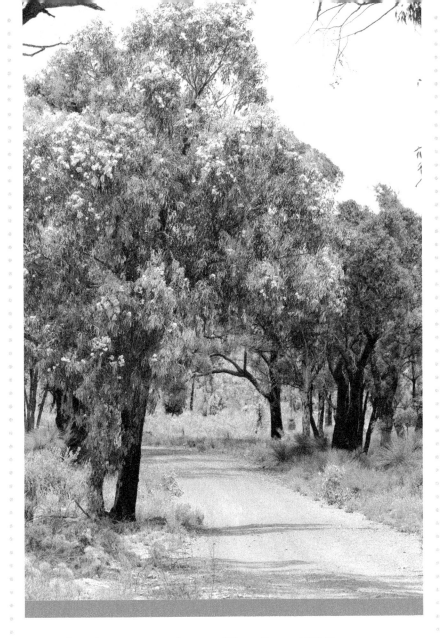

coastal and near-coastal areas (FloraBase, 2016).

Distribution Blackbutt is native to the south-west of Western Australia. It grows between Perth and Dongara and east as far as the Avon Wheatbelt (FloraBase, 2016).

Uses For the Noongar people's use of Eucalypts, see page 24.

Active Constituents For Eucalypts' active constituents, see page 24.

Eucalypts

The Eucalypts listed in this book were all used in similar ways by the Noongar people and share the same active constituents, as described below.

Parts Used
The leaves and gum.

Medicinal Uses
The leaves of all Eucalypts in the south-west of Western Australia were used crushed as antibacterial poultices for healing wounds. They were also used in steam pits and held, crushed, under the nose to relieve congestion due to colds and flu. The gum was ground and used as ointment for sores. It was also eaten to relieve dysentery (City of Joondalup, 2011; Cunningham, 1998).

Other Uses
The leaves of all Eucalypts in the south-west were used as bedding.

Active Constituents
Oil obtained from the leaves of all Eucalypt species contains 1,8-cineole

(eucalyptol), which has antibacterial, cough suppressant, expectorant, nasal decongestant and respiratory anti-inflammatory properties. The oil also contains the following active constituents, all of which have strong to mild antibacterial properties and some of which have antifungal properties: α-pinene, δ-limonene, α-terpineol, *p*-cymene, terpinen-4-ol, cuminal aldehyde, globulol, *p*-isoproplyphenol (australol) phenol, eudesmol and aromadendrene (Abbott & Abbott, 2015).

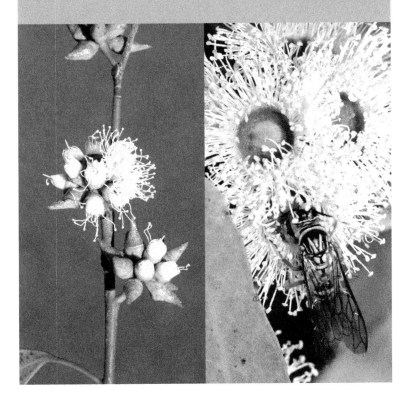

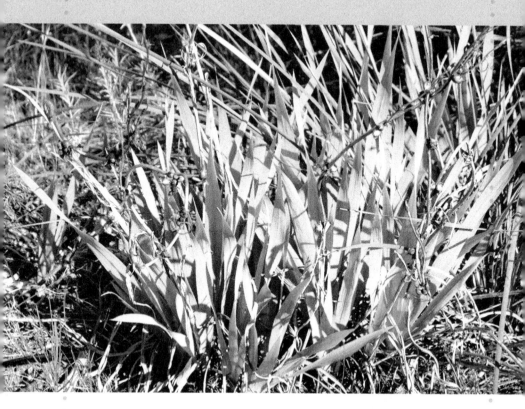

Family Haemodoraceae R.Br.

Botanical Name *Haemodorum spicatum* R.Br.

Common Name Bloodroot.

Noongar Names Born (northern part of south-west Western Australia), Koolung, Meen, Mardja (south-west Western Australia) and Matje (Abbott, 1983; Bennett, 1991).

Description Bloodroot is a grass-like shrub that grows to around 2 m high. It has long, slender, green leaves that grow each year to around 600 mm long. The leaves turn black as they age (SERCUL, 2014b). Bloodroot gets its name from the colour of the red, bulbous root, which was commonly eaten by Noongars. It is apparently quite spicy on the palate (Archer, 2016).

Habitat Bloodroot prefers sand, clay and laterite soils in wetland areas (Florabase, 2016).

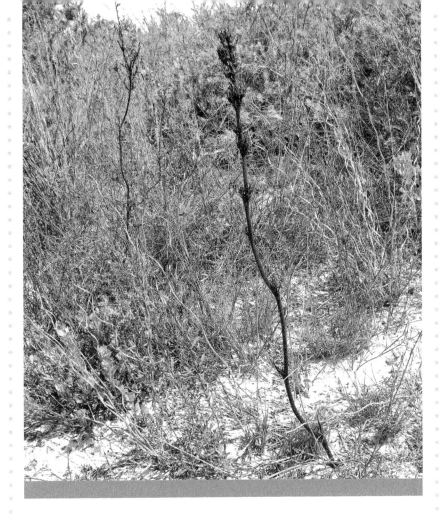

Distribution Bloodroot occurs in south-western Western Australia in coastal and near-coastal areas from Dongara to the east of Esperance (FloraBase, 2016).

Parts Used The roots and leaf bases.

Medicinal Uses The roots and leaf bases were roasted, pounded with clay from termites' nests and then eaten to stop diarrhoea in dysentery (Lassak & McCarthy, 2001). Decoctions of the bulbs (made by boiling them in water) were drunk to relieve lung congestion. The bulbs pounded into paste were rubbed into the body to treat arthritis.

Other Uses The bulbs were eaten, raw or roasted, as food (Lassak & McCarthy, 2001). The colour of the Bloodroot was extracted and used as a dye.

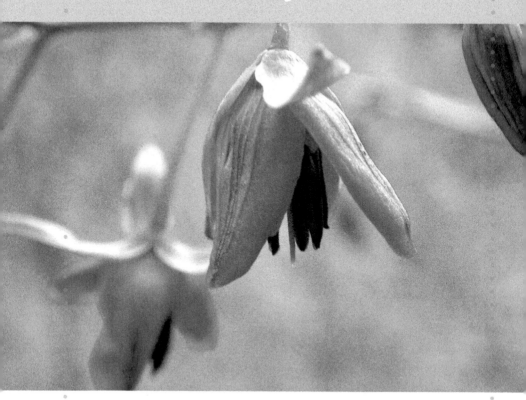

Botanical Name *Dianella revoluta* R.Br.

Common Names Blue Flax-lily, Blueberry Lily, Spreading Flax-lily and Black-anther Flax-lily.

Noongar Name Mangard.

Description Blue Flax-lily is a small, clumping, drought-resistant plant that grows to around 1 m tall and spreads to around 1.5 m. It has long, leafy, grass-like stems, which are glossy green and leathery in appearance. The plant produces small, bell-shaped, purple or blue flowers that are around 10 mm long. The flowers usually appear in late spring to summer (Kambarang to Birak). The fruits are globe-like and purple (SERCUL, 2014b).

Habitat Blue Flax-lily thrives in open forests, woodland and mallee areas in a variety of soils (FloraBase, 2016).

Family **Phormiaceae.**

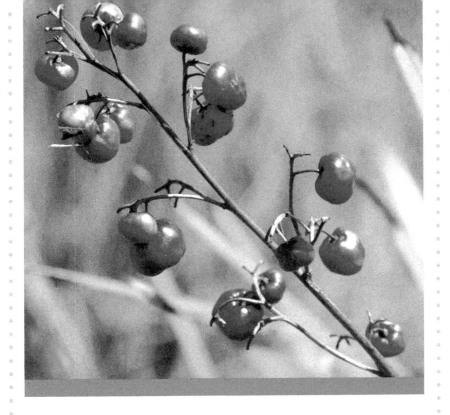

Distribution Blue Flax-lily is native to the south-west of Western Australia. It is also found in the southern reaches of South Australia, Victoria, New South Wales, Tasmania and south-east Queensland (Collis, 2007).

Parts Used The leaves, roots and fruits.

Medicinal Uses Decoctions of the leaves were taken internally to relieve headaches, while decoctions of the bulbous roots were drunk to treat colds.

Other Uses The fruits were eaten, raw or cooked. They have a sweet flavour that becomes nutty when the seeds are chewed. The roots, after pounding, were roasted and then eaten. The leaves were used to make string and cord for binding (SERCUL, 2014b).

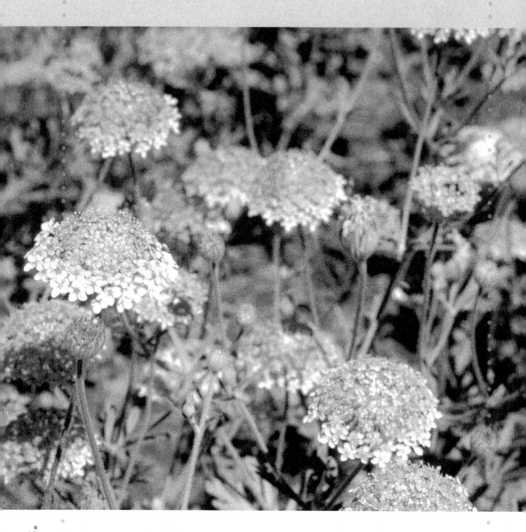

Botanical Name *Trachymene coerulea* Graham.

Common Names Blue Lace Flower and Rottnest Island Daisy.

Noongar Names Not known for this plant.

Description Blue Lace Flower is an annual or biennial herb and grows to about 0.2-1.0 m in height. The leaves are oval shaped and divided into segments. The flower stalks are hairy and around 200 mm-1m long. The flower heads are umbrella shaped, spreading to around 60 mm across (BGPA, 2012).

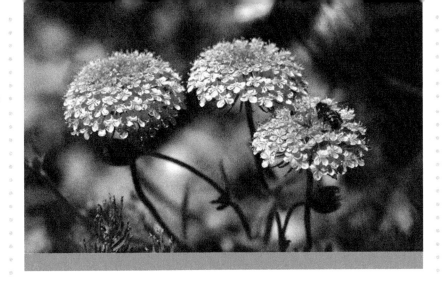

Habitat Blue Lace Flower thrives in sand over granite and limestone (FloraBase, 2016).

Distribution Blue Lace Flower is native to the south-west of Western Australia and grows mainly on the Swan Coastal Plain from Dongara to Augusta and on Rottnest and Garden islands (FloraBase, 2016).

Parts Used The bulbs and leaves.

Medicinal Uses The bulbs and leaves were mashed then rubbed into the body to relieve aches and pains. The leaves were also crushed and the vapours inhaled to treat headaches.

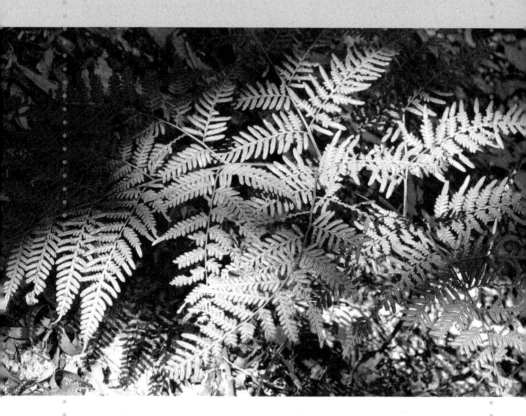

Family Dennstaedtiaceae Lotsy.

Botanical Name *Pteridium esculentum* (G.Forst.) Cockayne.

Common Names Bracken Fern, Bracken, Common Bracken (Bennett, 1991), Austral Fern and Austral Bracken.

Noongar Names Manya (Denmark area), Munda (Perth area), Moondan-gurnang (Abbott, 1983).

Other Aboriginal Names Gurgi and Eora (New South Wales).

Description Bracken Fern is a perennial (everlasting) plant that has an extensive, creeping, hairy rhizome-type root system, which allows it to spread. The stems grow up to 2.5 m long and are brown and stiff, bearing large, deeply divided, light green fronds that turn brown as they age (HerbiGuide, 2014).

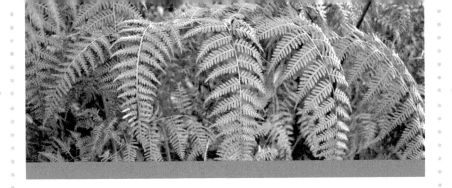

Habitat Bracken Fern likes laterite, gravel, white sand, red loam and brown clay. It inhabits moist, sandy areas, grows beside creeks and is prominent in Eucalypt forests (FloraBase, 2016).

Distribution Bracken Fern is found in coastal and near-coastal areas throughout Australia, except the Northern Territory. In Western Australia, it is found mostly in coastal areas from Geraldton to the South Australian border (FloraBase, 2016; Atlas of Living Australia, 2016).

Parts Used The leaves, stems, tips and roots.

Medicinal Uses Infusions of the crushed leaves were used externally as washes to relieve sores and rheumatic pain. They were also taken internally to treat intestinal worms, including tapeworms. Infusions of the leaves and stems were applied externally to relieve arthritis. Juice from the young stems and crushed leaves was rubbed into the skin to relieve insect and ant bites (Lassak & McCarthy, 2001).

Other Uses The fresh, unfolding tips and the horizontal rhizomes were eaten as food after extensive preparation. The roots are usually soaked in water for 24 hours then dried. The hairs were picked off, as they are an irritant (Daw, Walley & Keighery, 2011).

Active Constituents The whole plant contains condensed tannins as well as leucocyanidin. The leaves contain saponin pteridin, which is believed to kill intestinal worms (Lassak & McCarthy, 2001).

Botanical Name *Exocarpos sparteus* R.Br.

Common Names Broom Ballart and Native Cherry.

Noongar Names Djuk and Chuck (Abbott, 1983).

Description Broom Ballart grows 2–4 m tall as a shrub or small tree. Its leaves are small and fall early. The flower stalks are initially green, turning to scarlet later. The flowers are tiny and develop into edible fruits, with the seeds forming at the extreme ends (Archer, 2016).

Habitat Broom Ballart favours calcareous sand over limestone, although not exclusively. It is also found in inland mallee regions and where sandy loam overlies limestone (Archer, 2016).

Distribution Broom Ballart is particularly widespread in Australia, occurring throughout the mainland (NSWFO, 2016). In Western Australia, it is widespread along the coastline but is more sporadic inland. It is very prolific across the south-west from Shark Bay to Israelite Bay (Archer, 2016; FloraBase, 2016).

Parts Used The leaves and twigs.

Medicinal Uses The leaves and twigs were burnt to make smoke to repel insects. The leaves were crushed to make poultices, which were rubbed on the head to alleviate headaches.

Family Santalaceae R.Br.

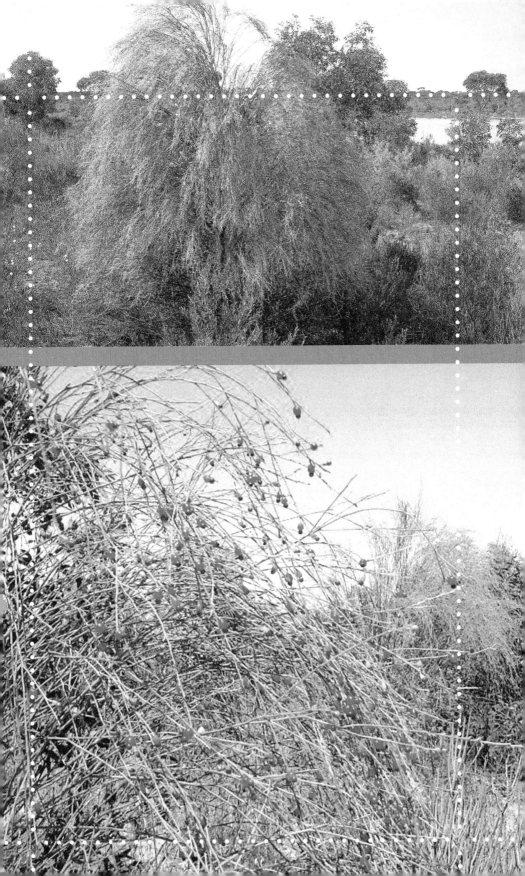

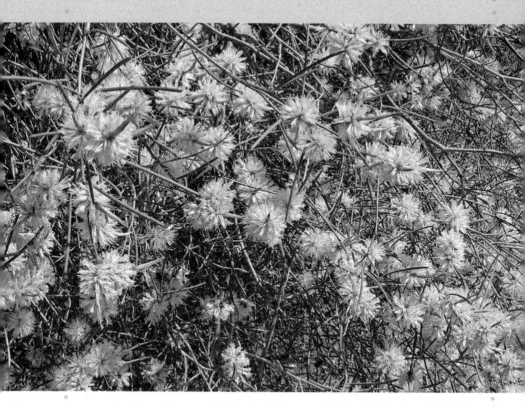

Family **Myrtaceae Juss.**

Botanical Name *Melaleuca uncinata* R.Br.

Common Names Broom Bush and Honey Myrtle.

Noongar Names Kwytyart and Yilberra (Abbott, 1983).

Description Broom Bush is a densely branching shrub that grows 500 mm–5.0 m tall. It has peeling, papery bark. The white-cream-yellow flowers appear from February to March (Bunuru) or from July to December (late Makuru to early Birak). The globular fruits appear during the summer months (Birak to early Bunuru) (Florabank, 2016).

Habitat Broom Bush grows in a variety of soils, including sand, clay and laterite soils. Habitats where it can be found include sandplains and wetlands (Florabase, 2016).

Distribution Broom Bush is native to the south-west of Western Australia and is widespread throughout inland areas

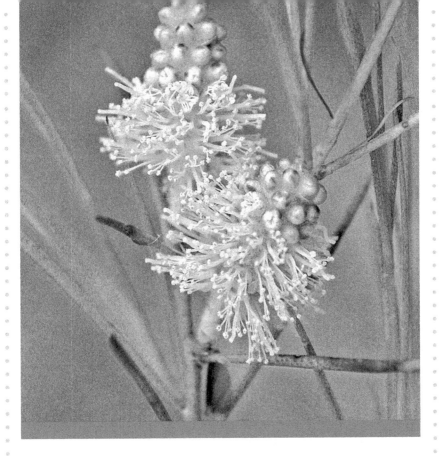

from Geraldton to Israelite Bay. It also occurs in the coastal areas of South Australia (Florabank, 2016; FloraBase, 2016).

Parts Used The whole plant.

Medicinal Uses Melaleucas have a strong aroma and were used to treat headaches, respiratory problems, coughs, stomach upsets and rheumatic aches and pains. The leaves were chewed to relieve respiratory complaints (Cribb & Cribb, 1983). Decoctions of the bark were used externally as washes to relieve sores, burns, skin infections and headaches. The whole plant was crushed and mixed with fat to make ointments or salves which were applied to treat muscular aches and arthritis.

Other Uses This plant was used by colonists to make brush fences.

Active Constituents For Melaleucas' active constituents, see page 83.

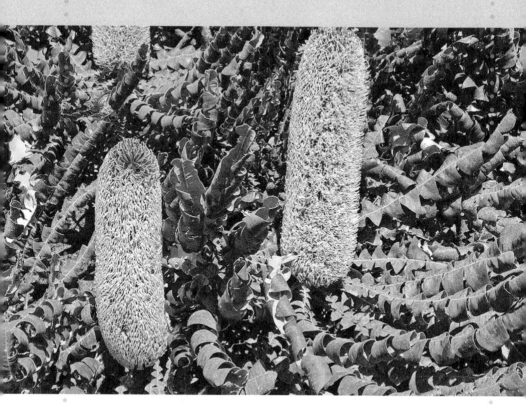

Botanical Name *Banksia grandis* Willd.

Common Names Bull Banksia, Giant Banksia and Mangite.

Noongar Names Mungite, Poolgarla (City of Joondalup, 2011), Mangij, Mungytch (Pibulmun for the flower) (Bourne, 2016) and Beera.

Description Bull Banksia grows as a shrub or tree 1.5–10 m in height. Its leaves grow up to 450 mm long and have triangular segments. The long, cylindrical flowers are yellow-green in colour. They appear from September to December (late Djilba to early Birak). Large cones appear after the flowers (ANPSA, 2016; FloraBase, 2016).

Habitat Bull Banksia prefers sand and laterite on coastal sandplains (FloraBase, 2016).

Family Proteaceae Juss.

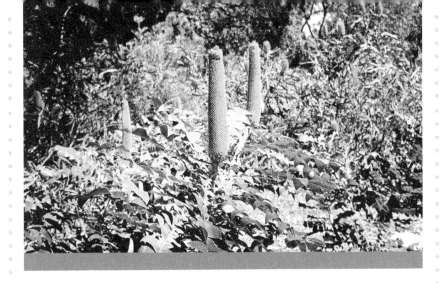

Distribution Bull Banksia occurs in coastal areas and inland from Jurien Bay to Albany. It can be seen to the east of Perth around York, Northam and Toodyay (FloraBase, 2016).

Parts Used The flowers.

Medicinal Uses For Banksias' medicinal uses, see page 16.

Other Uses The cones of Bull Banksia were used as fuel for fires and were wrapped in paperbark to carry fire from one camp to the next (Bourne, 2016). For Banksias' other uses, see page 16.

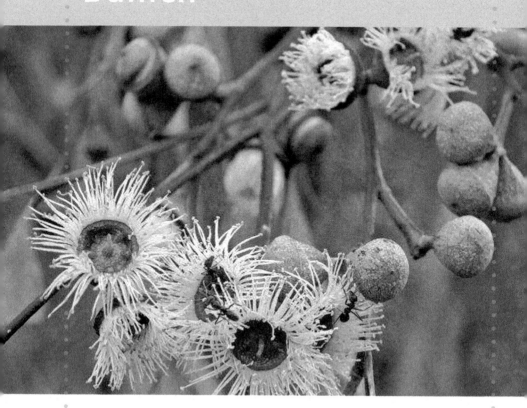

Botanical Name *Eucalyptus megacarpa* F.Muell.

Common Name Bullich.

Noongar Names Bullich (Abbott, 1983).

Description Bullich grows as either a tree to 35 m or as a smaller mallee to around 2 m. The bark is smooth and mottled. White flowers appear from mid autumn to late spring (Djeran to Kambarang) (FloraBase, 2016).

Habitat Bullich is found in sand or sandy loam over limestone in hilly areas, near swamps and streams (FloraBase, 2016).

Distribution Bullich is native to Western Australia and is scattered throughout the forests of the south-west of the state in coastal and near-coastal areas from Perth to Albany (FloraBase, 2016).

Family Myrtaceae Juss.

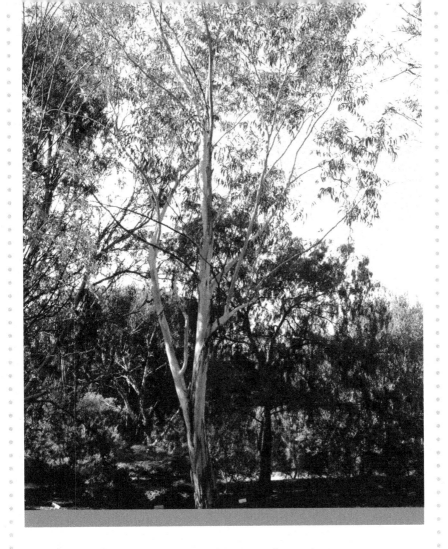

Uses For the Noongar people's use of Eucalypts, see page 24.

Active Constituents For Eucalypts' active constituents, see page 24.

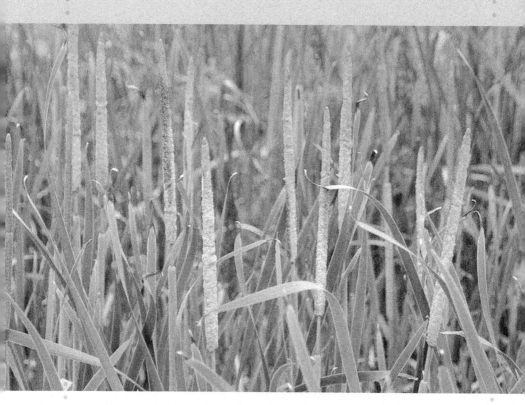

Botanical Name *Typha domingensis* Pers.

Common Names Bulrush, Reedmace and Narrow-leaved Cumbungi.

Noongar Names Yangeti, Yanget, Lirimbi, Yanjidi, Yunjeedie, Yunjid, Tanjil and Yandijut (Abbott, 1983; Bennett, 1991).

Other Aboriginal Names Cumbungi (New South Wales).

Description Bulrush is a water-loving plant that lives for several years. It grows to 3 m high. The rhizomes grow to 20 mm in diameter. The blade-like leaves grow to 2 m long and are around 20 mm wide. The flowers of both sexes grow on a single plant and are usually 120–400 mm long (Flora of Australia Online, 2016). The flowers grow on long stalks and are brownish in colour. They appear from May to September (late Djeran to Djilba) (FloraBase, 2016).

Family Typhaceae Juss.

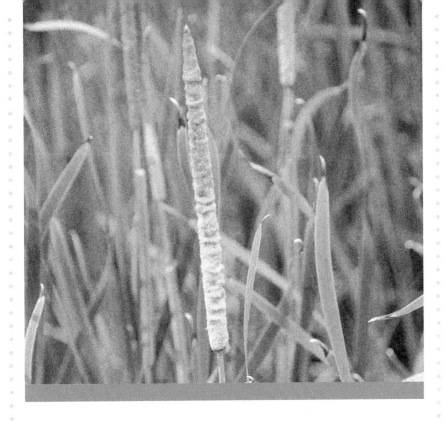

Habitat Bulrush loves clay and sand substrate. It grows beside freshwater swamps, creeks and rivers (FloraBase, 2016).

Distribution Bulrush is native to Western Australia but is found throughout Australia and in other countries. It is more prolific in the south-west of Western Australia.

Parts Used The leaves and roots.

Medicinal Uses The crushed female flowers of the Bulrush had medicinal uses as an antiseptic (Survival.org.au, 2011).

Other Uses The tuberous roots contain starch similar to that of sweet potatoes and were a good source of food for Noongars, who ate them raw or cooked. Shredding the leaves, drying them and weaving them into mats and baskets filled in many hours for Noongar women. When the plant was burnt, the smoke was a successful insect repellent (Survival. org.au, 2011).

Botanical Name *Eucalyptus burracoppinensis* Maiden & Blakely.

Common Name Burracoppin Mallee.

Noongar Name Muruk (City of Joondalup, 2011).

Description Burracoppin Mallee is drought resistant and grows to around 6 m in height. The bark is rough on the lower trunk, and there is smooth bark above. The leaves are mid green and lance shaped. The spiky flowers appear from August to November (Djilba to Kambarang) and are white-cream-yellow in colour (FloraBase, 2016).

Habitat Burracoppin Mallee grows best in sand, loam and pebbly soil in drier areas away from the coast (FloraBase, 2016).

Distribution Burracoppin Mallee is native to the south-west of Western Australia and is generally found in the Central Wheatbelt, the Merredin and Burracoppin area and south to Kulin (FloraBase, 2016).

Uses For the Noongar people's use of Eucalypts, see page 24.

Active Constituents For Eucalypts' active constituents, see page 24.

Family Myrtaceae Juss.

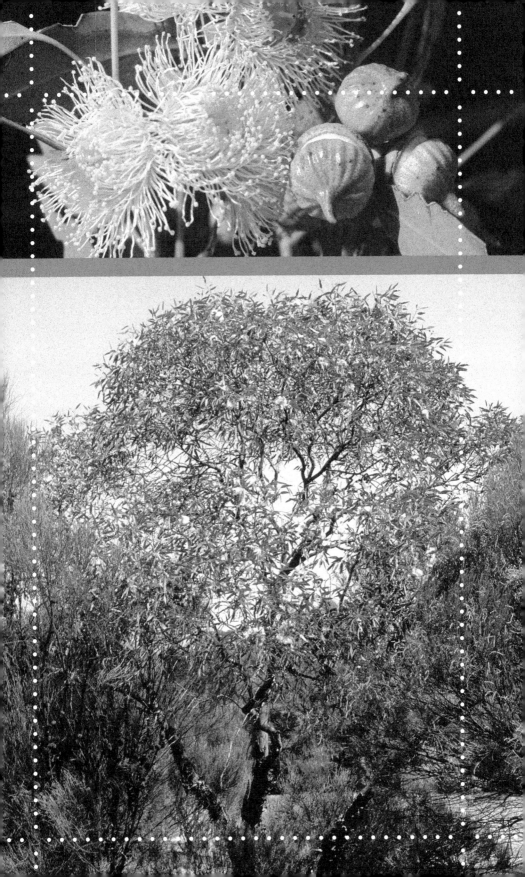

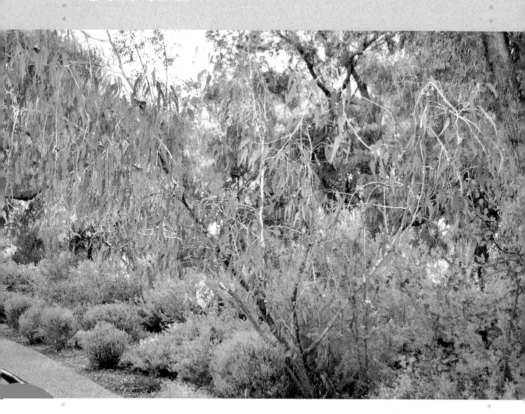

Family Myrtaceae Juss.

Botanical Name *Eucalyptus caesia* Benth.

Common Names Caesia, Gungurru and Silver Princess.

Noongar Names Gungurra, Gungunnu and Gungurru (Bennett, 1991).

Description Caesia grows as a small or large mallee 1.8–14 m high. The minni-ritchi bark, which looks like it is peeling off, is one of its main features, together with its beautiful pink to red flowers and the silver appearance of its stems. The leaves are blue-green in colour but because of their coating can appear whitish in bright sunlight (ANPSA, 2016). The flowers appear in winter and spring (Makuru to Kambarang).

Habitat Caesia prefers loam over granite outcrops but will grow in most soils (BGPA, 2015; FloraBase, 2016).

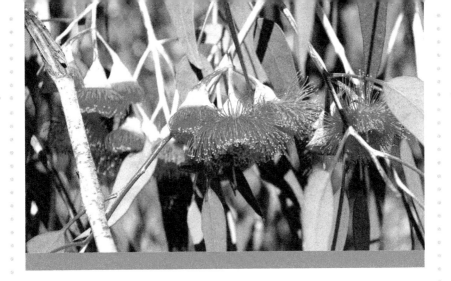

Distribution Caesia is native to the south-west of Western Australia and is scattered through the Central and Eastern wheatbelts east and north-east of Perth (FloraBase, 2016). Because it is a beautiful ornamental tree which tolerates sandy soils, it is found in gardens and parks all over the Perth greater metropolitan area.

Uses For the Noongar people's use of Eucalypts, see page 24.

Active Constituents For Eucalypts' active constituents, see page 24.

Camphor Myrtle

Botanical Names *Babingtonia camphorosmae* (Endl.) Lindl., formerly *Baeckea camphorosmae* Endl.

Common Names Camphor Myrtle and Eczema Plant.

Noongar Name Kurren.

Description Camphor Myrtle is a ground-hugging shrub growing to around 3 m high. It has quite small, almost oval leaves that are distributed evenly along its long stems. Its pink and white flowers appear from May to December (late Djeran to early Birak) or from January to February (late Birak to early Bunuru) (FloraBase, 2016).

Habitat Camphor Myrtle seems to prefer sand, as it grows in coastal and near-coastal areas (FloraBase, 2016).

Distribution Camphor Myrtle is native to the south-west of Western Australia and is found in coastal and near-coastal areas from the Geraldton Sandplains to Albany (FloraBase, 2016).

Parts Used The flowers, leaves and stems.

Medicinal Uses Infusions of the leaves were used to treat skin conditions such as eczema (Cunningham, 2005). The crushed leaves were waved under the nose and rubbed into the temples and behind the neck to treat headaches (Bindon, 1996). Decoctions of the leaves were taken internally to relieve upset stomachs and indigestion. The flowers, leaves and stems were crushed and mixed with fat to make ointments to treat skin conditions.

Family **Myrtaceae Juss.**

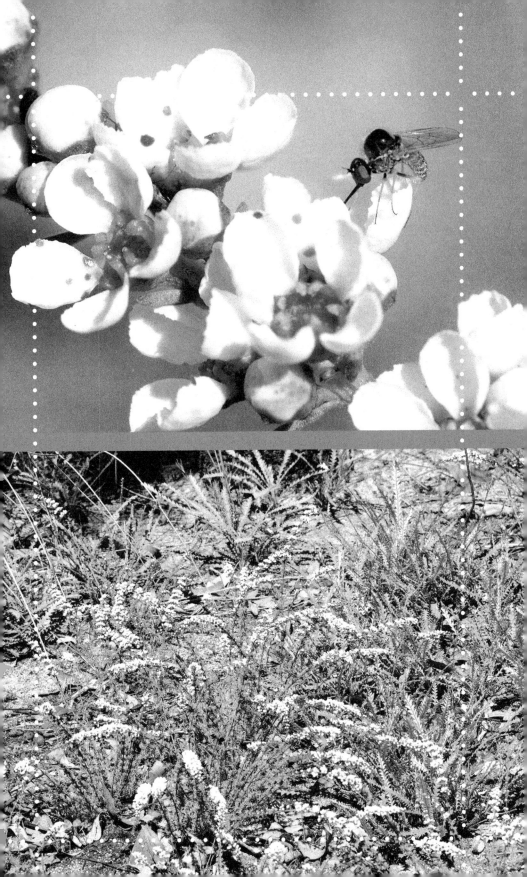

Caustic Weed

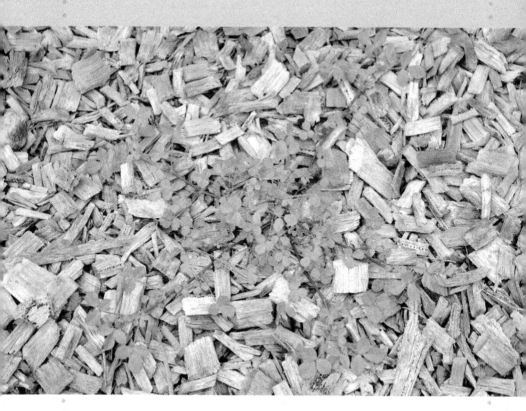

Botanical Name *Euphorbia drummondii* Boiss.

Common Names Caustic Weed, Caustic Creeper, Milk Plant, Pox Plant, Creeping Caustic and Mat Spurge.

Noongar Names Not known for this plant.

Other Aboriginal Names Ngama-ngama, Widda Pooloo, Piwi, Munya-munya, Yipi-kuyu-kuyu and Currawinya Clover.

Description Caustic Weed is a small, low-lying, short-lived herb that spreads to around 300 mm in diameter. It has a corrosive, milky sap when its red stems are broken. The small leaves are blue-green in colour. Small flowers appear from March to September (late Bunuru to Djilba) and can range from green-white to red-pink in colour (FloraBase, 2016).

Habitat Caustic Weed grows in disturbed ground and a range of soils, including clay, sand and stony hill soil

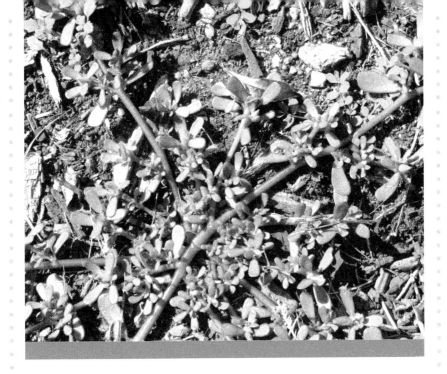

(FloraBase, 2016; Lassak & McCarthy, 2001).

Distribution Caustic Weed is quite prolific and is found throughout the Australian mainland from the tropics to the more temperate regions (Lassak & McCarthy, 2001).

Parts Used The sap, stems and leaves.

Medicinal Uses The milky sap was used as treatment for non-melanoma skin cancer, sores, cuts and scabies. Infusions of the stems and leaves were used by Aboriginals as cures for diarrhoea, dysentery and low fevers. Decoctions of the stems and leaves were used as washes for skin itches, sores, gonorrhoea and scabies (Lassak & McCarthy, 2001).

Other Uses Women used the sap to enlarge their breasts and to promote the flow of milk for breastfeeding (Peile, 1997).

Active Constituents The compound Ingenol-3-angelate, recently used in the treatment of skin cancers, can be isolated from various Euphorbia species, particularly from *E. peplus* and *E. drummondii Boiss.* Saponins and tannins are also found in *E. drummondii Boiss.* (Feng et al., 2011).

Coastal Pigface

Botanical Name *Carpobrotus virescens* (Haw.) Schwantes.

Common Name Coastal Pigface.

Noongar Names Bain (Coppin, 2008), Kolbolgo, Kolboje and Metjarak (Toodyay only) (Abbott, 1983).

Description Coastal Pigface is a ground-hugging succulent plant with a spread of around 3-4 m. The purple-pink flowers with white bases are around 60 mm in diameter. They appear from June to January (Makuru to Birak) (Archer, 2016; FloraBase, 2016). The fruits appear after the flowers fall off and are purplish red in colour (SERCUL, 2014b).

Habitat Coastal Pigface is found on sand dunes and coastal limestone cliffs (Archer, 2016; FloraBase, 2016).

Distribution Coastal Pigface is native to the south-west of Western Australia and can be seen along the coast from Geraldton to Israelite Bay (FloraBase, 2016).

Parts Used The fruits and leaves.

Medicinal Uses Infusions of the crushed leaves were used to treat diarrhoea, dysentery and stomach cramps, and as gargles to relieve sore throats, laryngitis and mild bacterial and fungal infections of the mouth. The juice of the leaves was used externally, much like Aloe Vera, to treat burns, abrasions, open cuts, grazes, mosquito bites and sunburn, and a variety of skin conditions, including fungal infections (such as ringworm and thrush), eczema, dermatitis, herpes, cold sores, cracked lips, chafing and allergies. The juice was also rubbed into the body to alleviate muscular aches and rheumatism (Coppin, 2008).

Other Uses The Noongar people ate the fruit, fresh or dried (Daw, Walley & Keighery, 2011).

Family Aizoaceae Martinov.

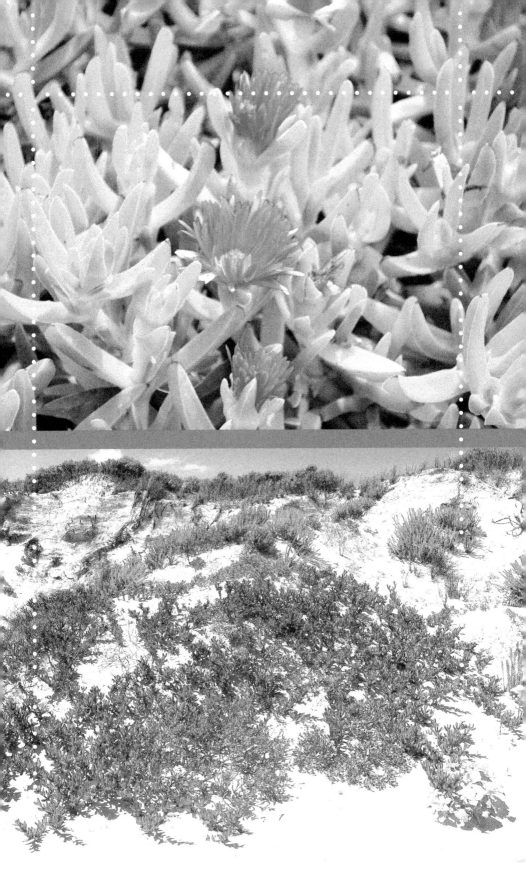

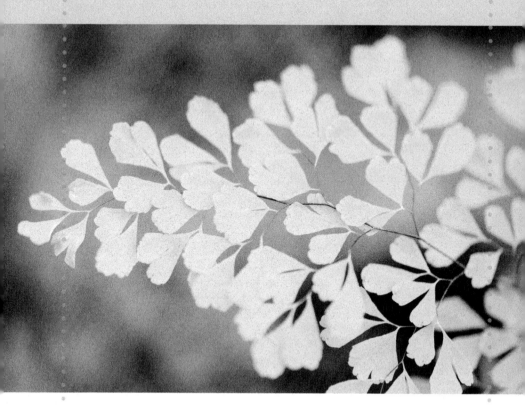

Family Pteridaceae E.D.M.Kirchn.

Botanical Name *Adiantum aethiopicum* L.

Common Names Common Maidenhair Fern and Small Maidenhair Fern.

Noongar Name Karbarra.

Description Common Maidenhair Fern is a rhizomatous, ground-hugging fern with a spreading nature. Its height varies from 100–600 mm. The fronds appear on dark brown stems. The small leaves have tiny spores, are almost circular and are bright green in colour (Lassak & McCarthy, 2001).

Habitat Common Maidenhair Fern prefers sand, clay, loam and laterite soils along damp banks in eucalypt forests (Florabase, 2016).

Distribution Common Maidenhair Fern is native to the south-west of Western Australia but is found in other parts of

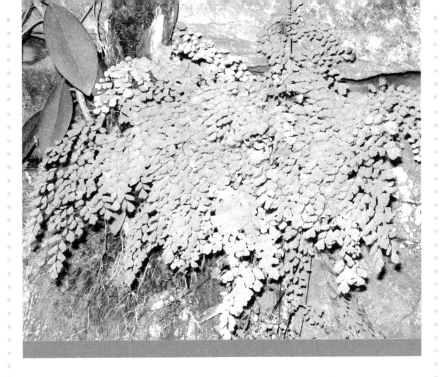

Australia and other countries. In Western Australia, it grows in coastal and near-coastal areas from just north of Perth to Albany (FloraBase, 2016).

Part Used The fronds.

Medicinal Uses Infusions of the fronds were taken internally in small amounts to treat chest infections or in larger amounts as emetics (Lassak & McCarthy, 2001). The fronds were crushed and the vapour inhaled to provide upper respiratory tract relief during colds, sinusitis and headaches.

Active Constituents The plant is thought to contain tannins but has not been properly investigated (Lassak & McCarthy, 2001).

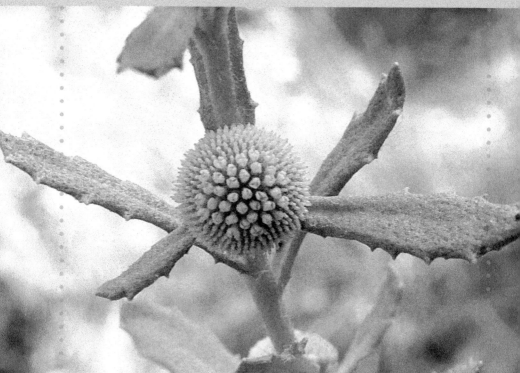

Family Asteraceae Bercht. & J.Presl.

Botanical Name *Centipeda cunninghamii* (DC.) A.Braun & Asch.

Common Names Common Sneezeweed, Common Sneezewood, Old Man Weed, Scentwood and Koona Puturku.

Noongar Names Not known for this plant.

Other Aboriginal Name Gukwonderuk (Koori).

Description Common Sneezeweed is a small, aromatic, semi-erect perennial herb that grows to approximately 300 mm high. It has stalkless, toothed, green leaves, which are tapered at both ends. Flowering in Western Australia occurs between spring and summer (late Djilba to early Bunuru) (Lazzak & McCarthy, 2001). The yellowish green fruits are spherical, with a bumpy appearance (TSU, 2016).

Habitat Common Sneezeweed grows in a variety of soils,

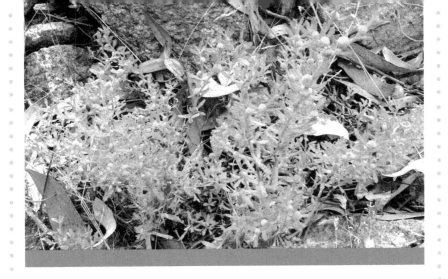

including alluvium, mud, sand and clay. It thrives beside rivers and salt lakes, in winter-wet depressions and on granite outcrops (FloraBase, 2016).

Distribution Common Sneezeweed is found throughout Australia. In the south-west of Western Australia it is found growing prolifically in coastal and near-coastal areas and more sporadically inland from Shark Bay to Israelite Bay.

Parts Used The whole plant.

Medicinal Uses Decoctions of the plant were used as eyewashes for the treatment of eye infections and sore eyes. In some parts of Australia, the black-coloured decoctions were used internally as tonics and treatment for general ill health, including tuberculosis, and externally as lotions to relieve skin infections. The leaves were sometimes put around the head to ease bad colds (Isaacs, 2009; Lassak & McCarthy, 2001).

Other Uses Aboriginal people of some inland groups put it around campsites at night; the plant's pungent odour kept ants away (Cribb & Cribb, 1983).

Active Constituents The essential oil contains chrysanthenyl and sabinyl acetates. Beattie, Waterman and Leach (2011) report that investigations on aqueous ethanolic extracts from this plant have confirmed its anti-inflammatory, antibacterial and antioxidant activity.

Couch Honeypot

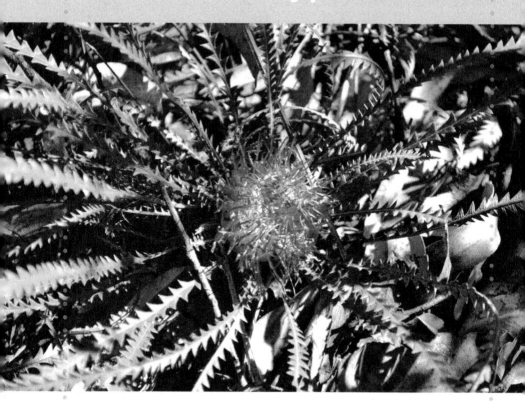

Family Proteaceae Juss.

Botanical Names *Banksia dallanneyi* A.R.Mast & K.R.Thiele, formerly *Dryandra lindleyana*.

Common Name Couch Honeypot.

Noongar Name Bullgalla.

Description Couch Honeypot is a ground-hugging Banksia that has a spreading nature. It has been found growing up to 3 m high. Its long, narrow, segmented leaves grow up to 200 mm in length. The flowers are globe shaped, orange-brown in colour and about 50 mm in diameter. They appear from June to October (Makuru to early Kambarang). The plant has the ability to regenerate after fires from underground lignotubers (ANPSA, 2016).

Habitat Couch Honeypot grows in a variety of soils, including sand, loam and laterite over granite and limestone.

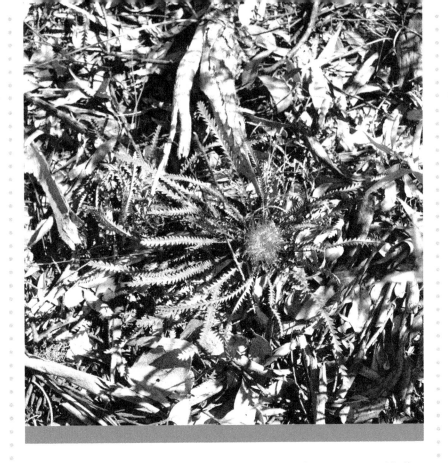

Habitats vary and include eucalypt forests, flat areas and hills (Florabase, 2016).

Distribution Couch Honeypot is native and specific to the south-west of Western Australia, occurring in coastal and near-coastal areas from Dongara to Esperance (FloraBase, 2016).

Uses For the Noongar people's use of Banksias, see page 16.

Desert Poplar

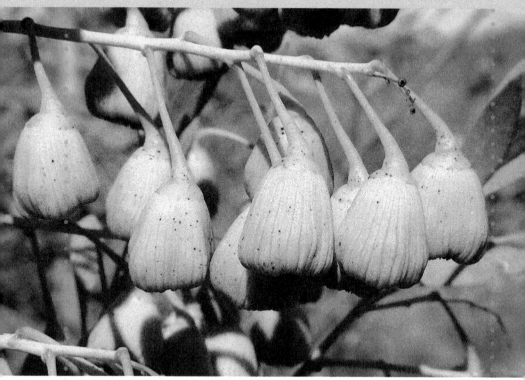

Family Gyrostemonaceae A.Juss.

Botanical Name *Codonocarpus cotinifolius* (Desf.) F.Muell.

Common Names Desert Poplar, Fire Tree, Bell Fruit Tree, Horseradish Tree, Quinine Tree, Medicine Tree, Firebush, Western Poplar and Toothache Tree (Lassak & McCarthy, 2001).

Noongar Names Not known for this plant.

Other Aboriginal Names Cucurdie, Cundilyong, Kandurangu (Meekathara), Garnduwangu (Yindjibarndi and Ngarluma) and Gandilangu (Wajarri).

Description Desert Poplar is a tall shrub or small tree that grows to around 6–10 m in height. The bark has dark red, yellow and green wavy lines. The pale green, oval-shaped leaves are tapered at the ends but broader near the tips. Yellow-green flowers appear from April to October (Djeran to early Kambarang). The bell-shaped fruits are green

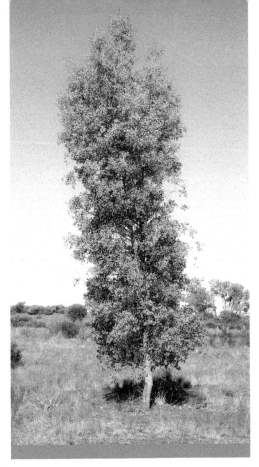

(FloraBase, 2016; Lassak & McCarthy, 2001).

Habitat Desert Poplar is found in red sand, loam and gravel in drier regions (FloraBase, 2016).

Distribution Desert Poplar occurs throughout Australia's drier regions, including those of the south-west, central and northern parts of Western Australia (FloraBase, 2016; Lassak & McCarthy, 2001).

Parts Used The roots, leaves, bark and shoots.

Medicinal Uses The roots, leaves and shoots were chewed and used as narcotics to ease toothaches and general pains. Decoctions of the bark, roots and stems were used externally as antiseptic washes for skin problems, such as eczema and sores, and as rubs to relieve rheumatic pain, colds, flu and fevers. An infusion of a combination of Desert Poplar (*Codonocarpus cotinifolius*) and Maroon bush (*Scaveola spinescens*) was thought to be a good treatment for cancer of various types (Lassak and McCarthy, 2001).

Active Constituents Lassak and McCarthy (2001) believe that the oil from the leaves contains benzyl cyanide and the sulphur containing glycoside cochlearin, but the active constituents are yet to be identified.

Botanical Names *Cassytha flava* Nees, *Cassytha glabella* R.Br., *Cassytha melantha* R.Br., *Cassytha pomiformis* Nees, *Cassytha racemosa* Nees.

Common Names Dodder Laurel, Tangled Dodder Laurel, Large Dodder Laurel and Devil's Twine.

Noongar Names Not known for these plants.

Description Dodder Laurels are leafless climbing plants that lack roots and bark. They are parasitic vines and climb over other plants, around which they take form. The light green stems are leafless. The fruits are oval-shaped globules and are almost transparent when they ripen (NQ Dry Tropics, 2015).

Habitat Dodder Laurels tolerate salt well and require only a good host plant (NQ Dry Tropics, 2015). They are found covering plants that like winter-wet areas, coastal limestone and laterite outcrops (FloraBase, 2016).

Distribution All of the Dodder Laurels listed above are native to the south-west of Western Australia and are found mainly in coastal areas from Geraldton to Esperance but have also been found in drier regions (FloraBase, 2016).

Parts Used The fruits.

Medicinal Uses Small quantities of the fruits were eaten as laxatives. The juice of the fruits was applied to cuts and sores to aid the healing process.

Family Lauraceae Juss.

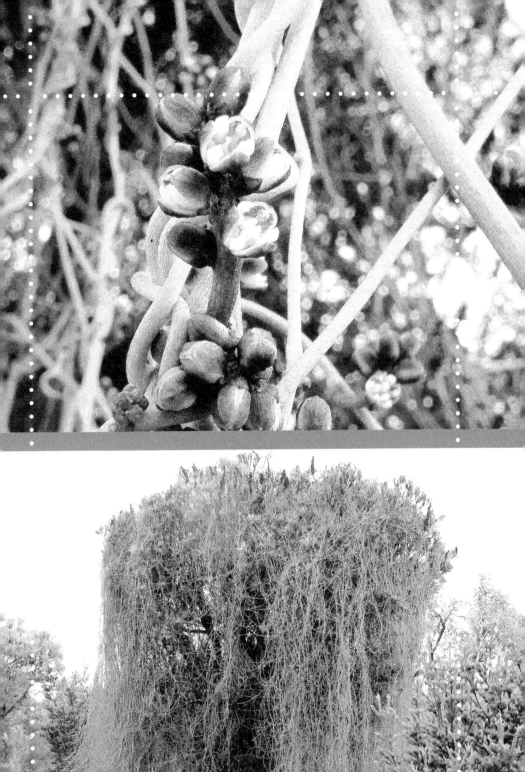
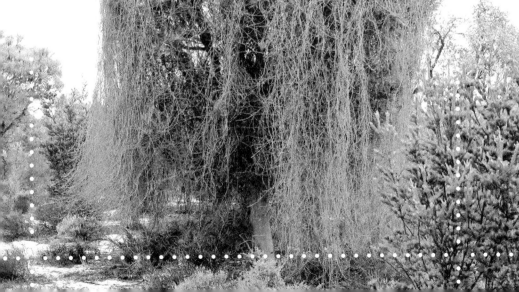

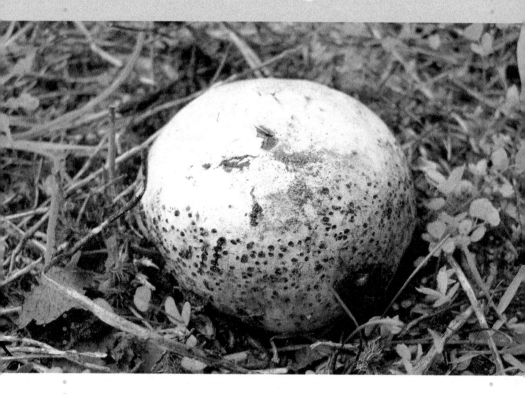

Family Sclerodermaceae.

Botanical Name *Pisolithus* sp.

Common Names Dog Poo Fungus, Horse Dung Fungus, Dead Man's Foot, Puffballs and Earth Balls.

Noongar Name Noomar (Noongar for fungi).

Description The fungi of this species appear as common brown puffballs, pale to dark mottled brown in colour. They can grow up to 200 mm in diameter and 200 mm tall. They break down into a mass of powdery spores (Bougher, 2009; Leithhead, 2016).

Habitat Dog Poo Fungi are very common in disturbed leaf litter, especially around Eucalypts (Readford, 2011).

Distribution Dog Poo Fungi are widespread throughout Australia and are also found worldwide. They are native to and very common in the south-west of Western Australia (Readford, 2011).

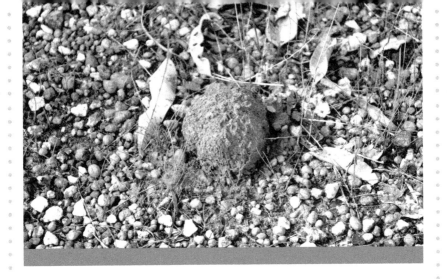

Parts Used The fruits.

Medicinal Uses The fruits were broken open and the spores rubbed into wounds and sores to prevent infection and promote healing.

Other Uses The young fruits were eaten by Noongars when food was scarce (ANBG, 2013). Robinson (2007) believes that a khaki dye made from the fruit of this fungus was used to dye military uniforms.

Active Constituents Bioactive components that have been identified by Ameri et al. (2011) include diterpenoids, triterpenoids, sesquiterpenoids and polysaccharides I, II, IIIA and IIIB, which they found to be effective against strains of methicillin-resistant *Staphylococcus aureus* (Golden Staphylococcus).

Caution

Bougher (2009) warns that a licence is needed to collect fungi on public land in Western Australia as fungi are a protected species.

Botanical Name *Alyxia buxifolia* R.Br.

Common Names Dysentery Bush, Heath Box, Sea Box, Tonga Bean Wood and Camel Bush (Bennett, 1991).

Noongar Names Not known for this plant.

Description Dysentery Bush is a shrub that can grow to around 3 m in height. It has dark green, oval-shaped leaves and white-cream or cream-orange, tubular flowers, which have a star-like appearance when viewed end on. The flowers usually appear from May to December (late Djeran to early Birak). The small, globular fruits are red when mature and are common throughout summer (Birak to early Bunuru) (Archer, 2016; FloraBase, 2016).

Habitat Dysentery Bush has no preference for soil type (Archer, 2016; FloraBase, 2016).

Distribution Dysentery Bush grows across southern Australia on or near the coast. It is found throughout the south-west of Western Australia from Jurien Bay to Esperance (Archer, 2016; FloraBase, 2016).

Parts Used The bark.

Medicinal Uses Decoctions of the crushed bark were drunk to treat diarrhoea and dysentery (Lassak & McCarthy, 2001).

Family Apocynaceae Juss.

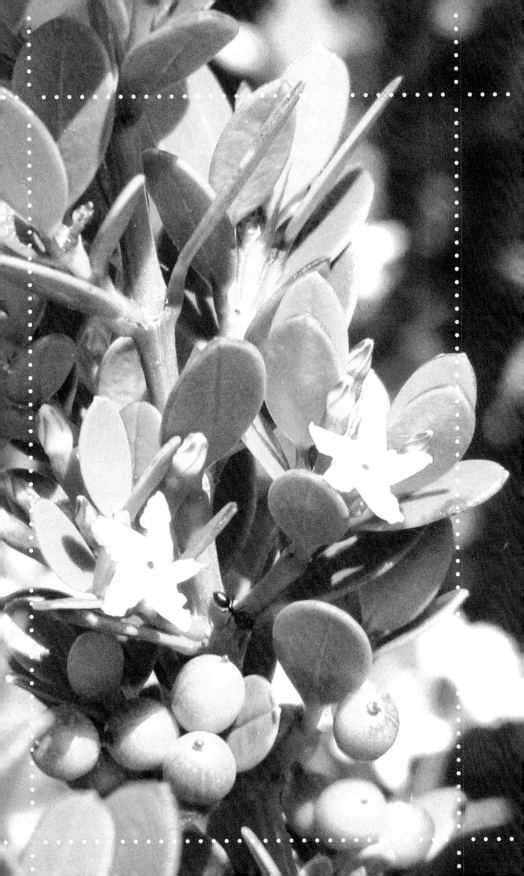

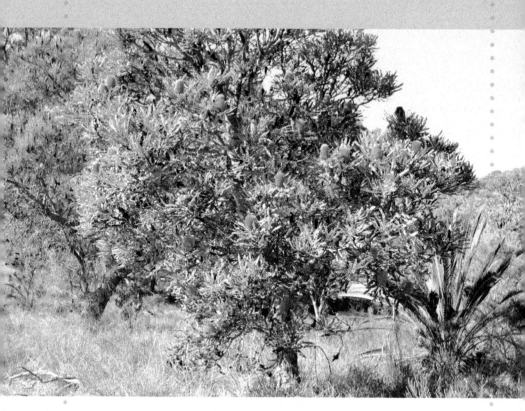

Botanical Name *Banksia menziesii* R.Br.

Common Name Firewood Banksia.

Noongar Name Bulgalla (City of Joondalup, 2011).

Description Firewood Banksia grows to around 7 m in height but may be a dwarf form, growing only to around 1 m in some areas where the soil is poor. The dull green leaves are serrated and oblong in shape. The red, pink or yellow flowers appear in autumn and winter (late Bunuru to early Djilba). Some flowers appear two coloured. The tree has a lignotuber, which allows it to regrow after a bushfire (ANPSA, 2016; FloraBase, 2016).

Habitat Firewood Banksia prefers sand near the coast (FloraBase, 2016).

Family Proteaceae Juss.

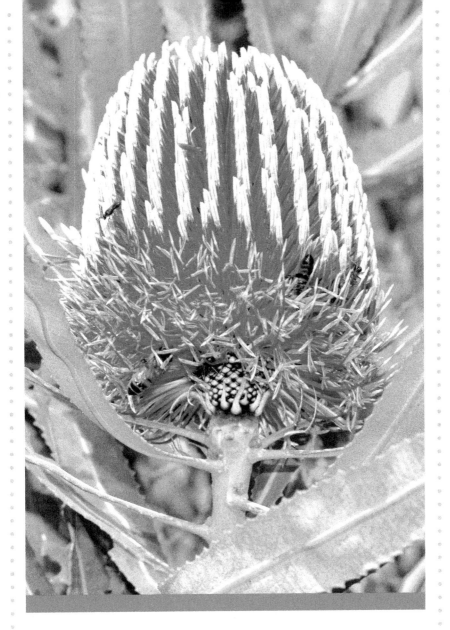

Distribution Firewood Banksia is native to the south-west of Western Australia and is found from the Murchison River to Busselton. It grows quite prolifically on the Perth and Geraldton sandplains and is also found in the Avon Wheatbelt and on the Dandaragan Plateau (FloraBase, 2016).

Uses For the Noongar people's use of Banksias, see page 16.

Flannel Bush

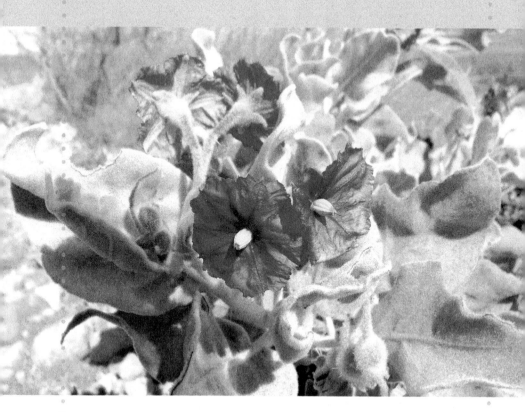

Botanical Name *Solanum lasiophyllum* Poir.

Common Names Flannel Bush and Native Tomato.

Noongar Name Grun Grun.

Other Aboriginal Names Pulgatura, Mindjulu and Taura (Bennett, 1991).

Description Flannel Bush is a prickly, bushy shrub that grows to 2 m high. It has round or broadly oval-shaped leaves that grow up to 50 mm long. The leaves are hairy on both sides. The purple-violet flowers appear in January (late Birak) or from April to October (Djeran to early Kambarang) (FloraBase, 2016; Lassak & McCarthy, 2001). Plant Broome (2016) describes the fruits as 'hard inedible drupes, fully enclosed by prickly bracts full of small brown/black seeds'.

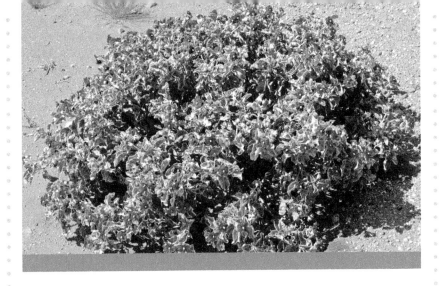

Habitat Flannel Bush occurs in a variety of soils, including sand and clay (FloraBase, 2016). It is sometimes found on stony rises (eFloraSA, 2013).

Distribution Flannel Bush grows all over Western Australia, except in the far north and far south (FloraBase, 2016). It is also found in parts of the Northern Territory and South Australia (eFloraSA, 2013).

Parts Used The roots.

Medicinal Uses Decoctions of the crushed roots were applied as poultices to leg swellings (Lassak & McCarthy, 2001).

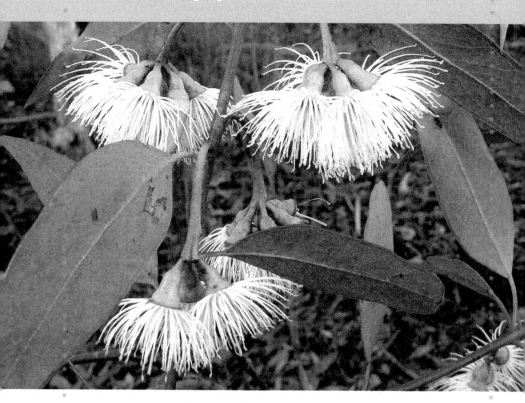

Botanical Name *Eucalyptus occidentalis* Endl.

Common Name Flat-topped Yate.

Noongar Name Mo (Abbott, 1983).

Description Flat-topped Yate commonly grows as a mallee near the coast, seldom reaching more than 15 m in height. It is usually a taller, single-trunked tree inland, reaching up to 25 m in height. The bark is rough, fibrous and flaky on the trunk but smooth on the higher branches (Archer, 2016). The leaves are eliptical or oval and are a dull grey-green colour (Eucalink, 2004). The cream or white flowers bloom from September to December (late Djilba to early Birak) or from January to May (late Birak to Djeran) (FloraBase, 2016).

Habitat Flat-topped Yate prefers sand or clay type soils in wetter areas near lakes and rivers (FloraBase, 2016).

Family Myrtaceae Juss.

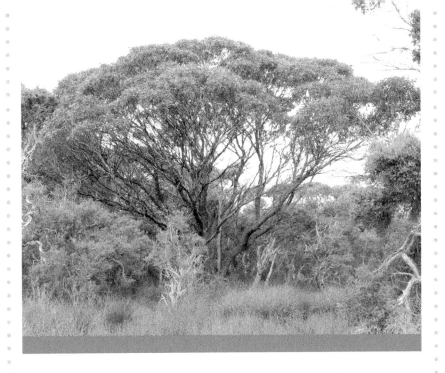

Distribution Flat-topped Yate is native to Western Australia and is scattered throughout the coastal areas of the southern region east from Denmark and Albany to Israelite Bay near the South Australian border plus inland as far north as the southern reaches of the Kalgoorlie and Coolgardie (FloraBase, 2016).

Parts Used The leaves, gum and wood.

Medicinal Uses For Eucalypts' medicinal uses, see page 24.

Other Uses Flat-topped Yate is fire resistant and saline tolerant and is often used by farmers in the south-west of Western Australia for windbreaks. The timber makes good poles and fence posts (Archer, 2016).

Active Constituents For Eucalypts' active constituents, see page 24.

Flooded Gum

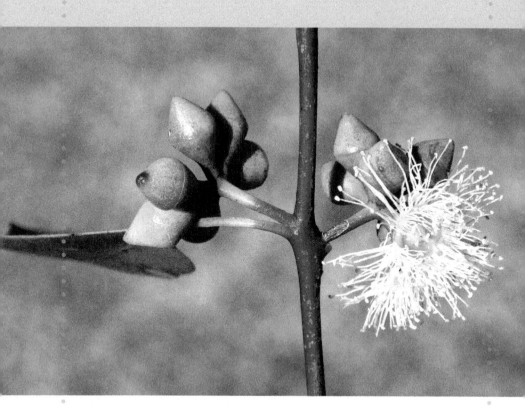

Botanical Name *Eucalyptus rudis* subsp. *rudis* Endl.

Common Names Flooded Gum, Blue Gum, Desert Gum, River Gum and Swamp Gum (Bennett, 1991).

Noongar Names Moich, Moitch, Kulurda, Gooloorto, Koolert, Moja, Gulurto (City of Joondalup, 2011), Colaille and Gulli (Abbott, 1983).

Description Flooded Gum is a Eucalypt that grows between 5 and 20 m tall depending on the conditions. It has rough, fibrous, dark grey bark on the trunk, with smooth, cream and pale grey bark on the higher branches. The leaves are broad and lance shaped, dull grey-green to bluish green, and around 120 mm long and 30 mm wide. The flowers are white and appear from July to September (late Makuru to Djilba). The fruits (gumnuts) are green and bell shaped (Bennett, 2016; FloraBase, 2016).

Family Myrtaceae Juss.

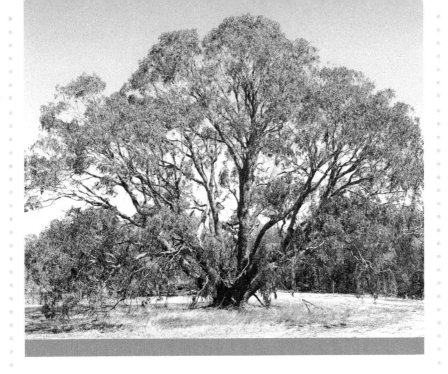

Habitat Flooded Gum prefers sand in wetter areas (FloraBase, 2016).

Distribution In Western Australia, Flooded Gum is found in coastal and near-coastal areas from Kalbarri to Bremer Bay (FloraBase, 2016).

Parts Used The leaves and gum.

Medicinal Uses For Eucalypts' medicinal uses, see page 24.

Other Uses Noongars used to eat the sugary substance (manna) on the leaves of the Flooded Gum which is produced by mites that live at the base of the leaves (City of Joondalup, 2011).

Active Constituents For Eucalypts' active constituents, see page 24.

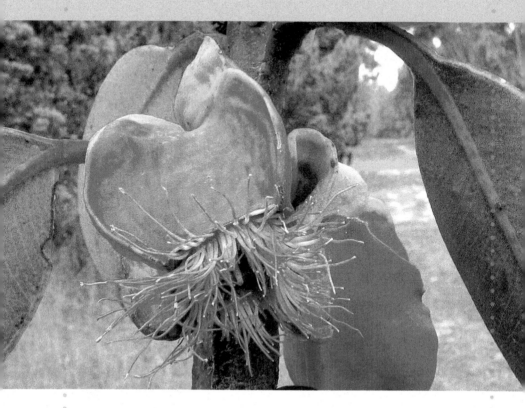

Botanical Name *Eucalyptus tetraptera* Turcz.

Common Names Four-winged Mallee and Square-fruited Mallee.

Noongar Names Not known for this tree.

Description Four-winged Mallee is a straggly, multi-trunked tree that grows to 3 m in height. The bark is smooth throughout the branches and grey in colour. The leaves when they first form are narrow or oval and dull grey-green but become glossy green later. The flowers bloom from June to December (Makuru to early Birak). The fruits or seed capsules are square and bright red and look like they have four wings – hence the common name (Archer, 2016; EucaLink, 2004).

Family Myrtaceae Juss.

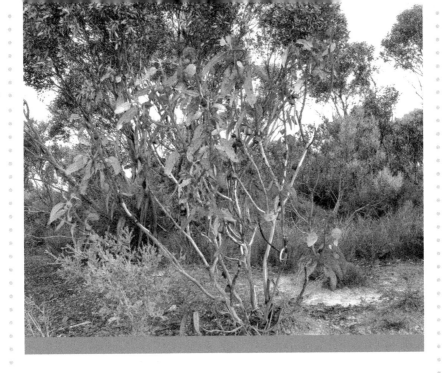

Habitat Four-winged Mallee grows in white and grey sand over gravel on coastal and subcoastal sandplains and granite outcrops (FloraBase, 2016).

Distribution Four-winged Mallee is native to Western Australia and is found in southern coastal and subcoastal areas from Albany to Israelite Bay (FloraBase, 2016).

Uses For the Noongar people's use of Eucalypts, see page 24.

Active Constituents For Eucalypts' active constituents, see page 24.

Botanical Name *Eucalyptus salubris* F.Muell.

Common Name Gimlet.

Noongar Names Nardarak, Gnardarup and Ngarrip (WNRM, 2009).

Description Gimlet is usually a small- to medium-sized Eucalypt tree that grows to around 15 m high, but some have been recorded as tall as 49 m (Cunningham, 1998). The trunk and upper limbs are grooved and are copper in colour. The narrow, lance-like, glossy green leaves are tapered at the bases. White-cream flowers appear from September to March (late Djilba to Bunuru) (Eucalink, 2004; FloraBase, 2016).

Habitat Gimlet is found in sandy clay, loam and clayey loam in drier areas, on plains and slopes (FloraBase, 2016).

Distribution Gimlet is sparse around the Perth area, as it prefers drier parts of the south-west. Its distribution ranges from Geraldton to Esperance and to the edge of the Nullarbor Plain beyond Kalgoorlie (FloraBase, 2016).

Uses For the Noongar people's use of Eucalypts, see page 24.

Active Constituents For Eucalypts' active constituents, see page 24.

Family **Myrtaceae Juss.**

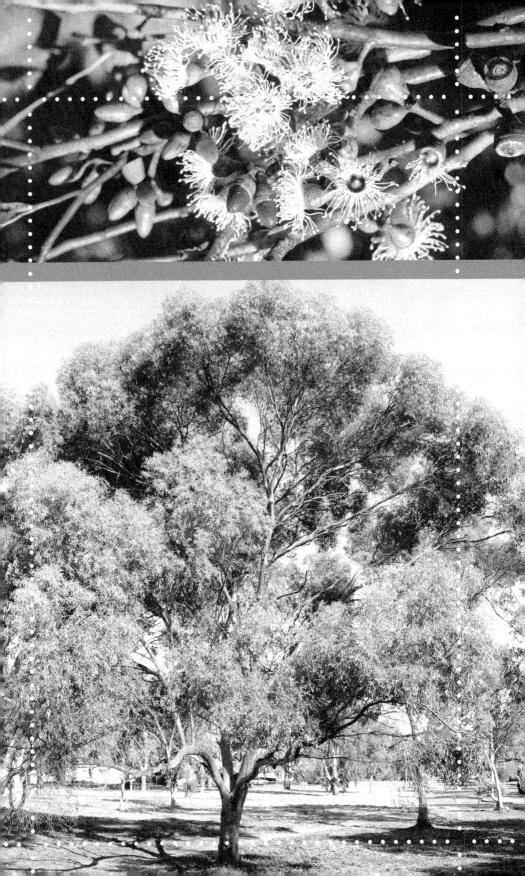

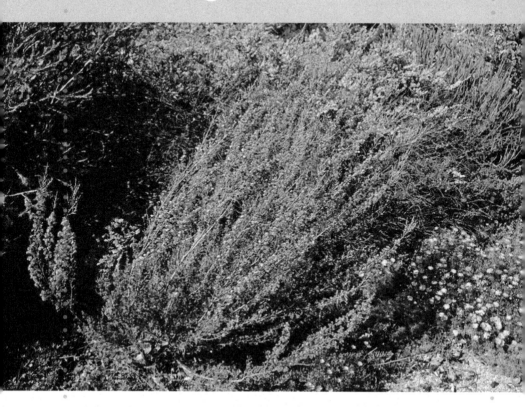

Botanical Name *Kunzea preissiana* Schauer.

Common Name Glowing Kunzea.

Noongar Name Kondill.

Description Glowing Kunzea is a spreading shrub that grows to around 2 m high. The thin stems of this plant have rough bark. The needle-like, green leaves are only about 20 mm long. The pink to pink-purple flowers have five petals and appear from August to October (Djilba to early Kambarang) (FloraBase, 2016).

Habitat Glowing Kunzea prefers sand and gravelly laterite (FloraBase, 2016).

Family Myrtaceae Juss.

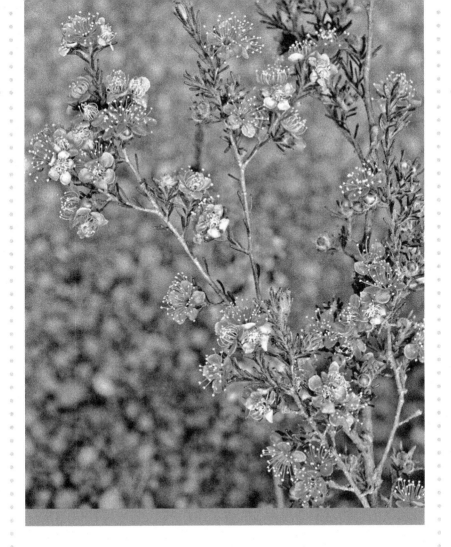

Distribution Glowing Kunzea is native to the south-west of Western Australia and is found from Perth to beyond Esperance, and inland in the Avon Wheatbelt and Eastern Mallee (FloraBase, 2016).

Parts Used The leaves and flowers.

Medicinal Uses The leaves and flowers were crushed and made into poultices which were applied to the body to relieve joint and muscle pains associated with arthritis and flu and to the head to ease nervous tension, stress and mild anxiety.

Botanical Name *Melaleuca radula* Lindl.

Common Name Graceful Honeymyrtle.

Noongar Name Moorngan.

Description Graceful Honeymyrtle is a shrub that ranges from 300 mm–2.4 m in height. The leaves are narrow, elliptical, aromatic and about 40 mm long. Purple, pink or white spiky flowers appear in winter and spring (Makuru to Kambarang). It produces small, purple, berry-like fruits (FloraBase, 2016).

Habitat Graceful Honeymyrtle grows in sand and gravelly soil over granite and laterite. More often than not it is found beside watercourses (FloraBase, 2016).

Distribution Graceful Honeymyrtle is endemic to the south-west of Western Australia. It is found from the Geraldton Sandplains to Perth and beyond the Avon Wheatbelt and Kalgoorlie (FloraBase, 2016).

Parts Used The leaves.

Medicinal Uses Decoctions of the leaves were used as antiseptic mouthwashes to treat sore gums and as external washes for sores and other skin problems; taken internally, they were used to treat upset stomachs and indigestion. Young leaves were chewed to relieve headaches and other ailments.

Active Constituents For Melaleucas' active constituents, see page opposite.

Family Myrtaceae Juss.

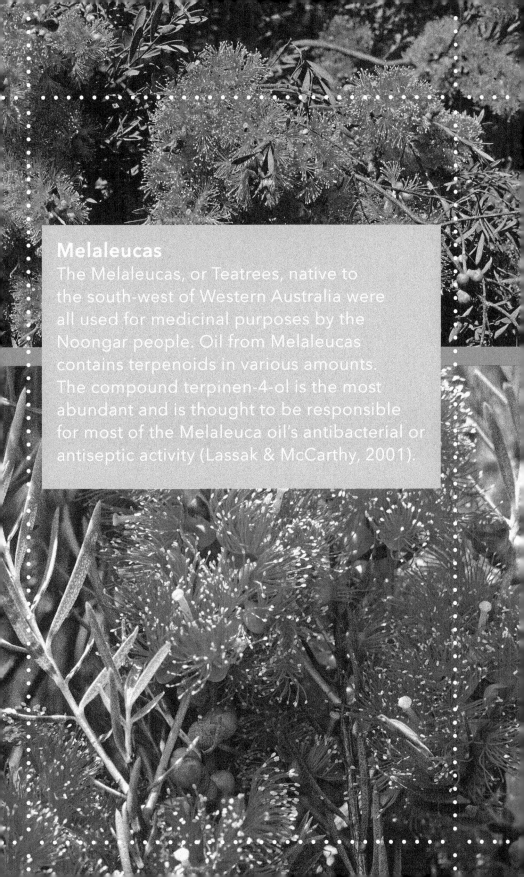

Melaleucas

The Melaleucas, or Teatrees, native to the south-west of Western Australia were all used for medicinal purposes by the Noongar people. Oil from Melaleucas contains terpenoids in various amounts. The compound terpinen-4-ol is the most abundant and is thought to be responsible for most of the Melaleuca oil's antibacterial or antiseptic activity (Lassak & McCarthy, 2001).

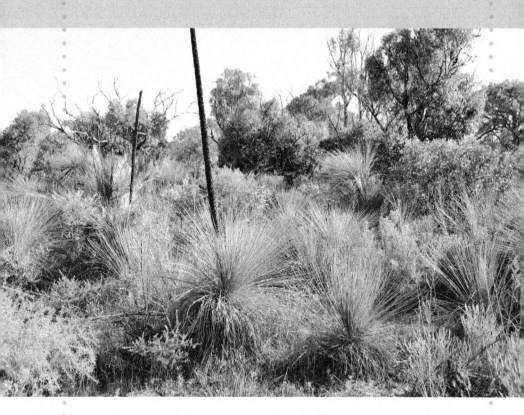

Family Xanthorrhoeaceae Dumort.

Botanical Name *Xanthorrhoea preissii* Endl.

Common Name Grass Tree.

Noongar Names Balga, Baaluk, Balgarr, Ballak, Balligar, Balluk, Baluk, Barar, Barlock, Barro, Beara, Paaluk and Paluk (Abbott, 1983).

Description Grass Trees can grow to 3 m tall. The thin, grass-like leaves that sprout from the top of the plant may reach 2.5 m in length. The white-cream flowers are produced from June to December (Makuru to early Birak) and protrude like spears from the top of the plant. The flowers turn brown after they have been on the tree for a while (FloraBase, 2016; FQPB, 2011).

Habitat Grass Trees grow in a variety of soils, including sand, loam and gravel (FloraBase, 2016).

Distribution Grass Trees occur throughout the south-west of Western Australia, on the coastal plain near watercourses from Geraldton to beyond Albany (FloraBase, 2016).

Parts Used The resin, pulp from inside the top of the trunk, shoots and flowers.

Medicinal Uses The gum is a normative and was chewed to relieve both diarrhoea and constipation. The pulp from the inside of the top of the tree was eaten to relieve upset stomachs. The smoke from burning the resin was inhaled to relieve sinusitis (City of Joondalup, 2011).

Other Uses Women were able to use the resin to start fires, as it is highly flammable. The resin was also used as a binding agent like cement – for example, to attach stone spearheads to wooden spear shafts. The glue was made by crushing the resin with charcoal and kangaroo droppings in a heated stone pot until molten. Grass Tree resin also worked as a tanning agent. Lumps were dissolved in water in a rock hole heated by hot stones, then the scraped and softened hides of kangaroos and possums were soaked in it. The skins were used as clothes, blankets and carry-bags (City of Joondalup, 2011).

The flower spikes were used as fishing spears, as torches to carry fire from one camp to the next and to spark fires by friction (City of Joondalup, 2011). Infusions of the flowers made sweet-tasting drinks. The flowers were also used as compasses: the buds open in conjunction with the sun's arc to enable direction calculation (Gardening Australia, 2011).

The young leaf shoots and the centre of the tree were eaten, as were the grubs that often inhabit the roots. The soft, white, powdery material inside the top of the trunk was squeezed like a sponge, and the white, milky liquid that emerges was used to quench thirst when drinking water was scarce.

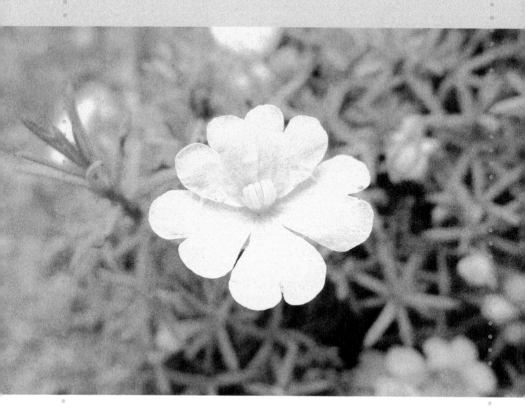

Family Dilleniaceae Salisb.

Botanical Name *Hibbertia glomerosa* (Benth.) F.Muell.

Common Name Guinea Flower.

Noongar Name Ballyion (Bourne, 2016).

Description Guinea Flower is a shrub that grows 600 mm–2 m high. It has small, slightly ovate leaves around 40 mm long. Its bright yellow, buttercup-like flowers have five petals and appear from July to November (late Makuru to Kambarang) (FloraBase, 2016).

Habitat Guinea Flower grows in a variety of soils, including sand, sandy clay, brown loam, gravel and laterite. It is found on sandplains, outcrops, rocky hills and the edges of claypans (FloraBase, 2016).

Distribution Guinea Flower is native to the south-west of Western Australia. It is found from the Geraldton Sandplains

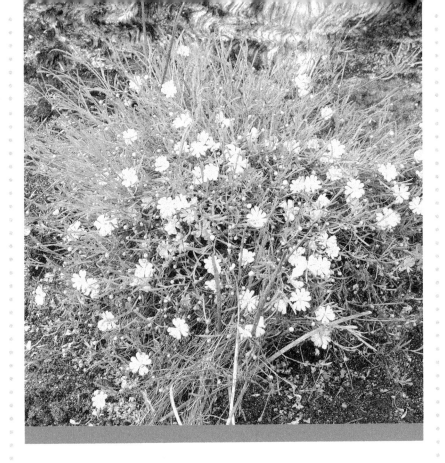

near the coast and inland to Denmark and as far east as Kalgoorlie (FloraBase, 2016).

Parts Used The leaves.

Medicinal Uses The leaves were crushed and used as antiseptic poultices applied to open wounds. Noongars used paperbark as bandages to keep the leaves in place (Bourne, 2016).

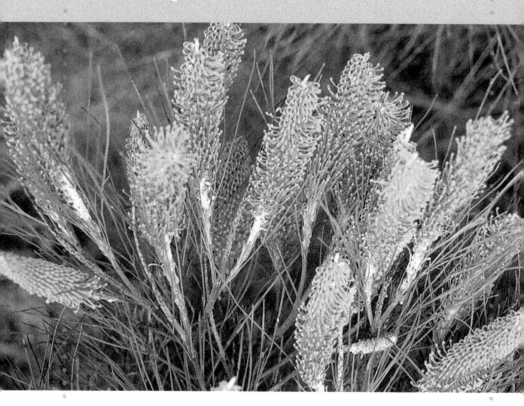

Family Proteaceae Juss.

Botanical Name *Grevillea juncifolia* Hook.

Common Names Honeysuckle Grevillea, Rush-leaved Grevillea and Spider Flower.

Noongar Names Moncart and Paarluc.

Description Honeysuckle Grevillea is an evergreen shrub or tree that grows from 4–7 m high depending on the conditions. The grey leaves are long and thin, with fine hairs on the surface. The bright yellow-orange, spider-like flowers are seen at various times of the year, in January (late Birak), from March to May (late Bunuru to Djeran) or from July to November (late Makuru to Kambarang) (Australian Native Plants Society, 2016).

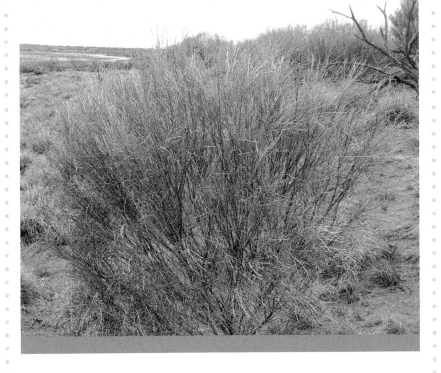

Habitat Honeysuckle Grevillea is found in rocky, stony and gravelly soil and sand among low trees and in shrubland (Australian Native Plants Society, 2016).

Distribution Honeysuckle Grevillea is native to the drier areas of Australia, except Victoria and Tasmania (Atlas of Living Australia, 2016). In the south-west, it is native to the drier areas from Geraldton to Perth and has been seen beyond Newman, Wiluna and Kalgoorlie (FloraBase, 2016). Because of its beautiful flowers, it is a prominent feature in parks and gardens around Perth.

Parts Used The bark.

Medicinal Uses The bark of the Honeysuckle Grevillea was burnt and the ash rubbed on sores, either as is or chewed, to encourage healing (Peile, 1997).

Illyarrie

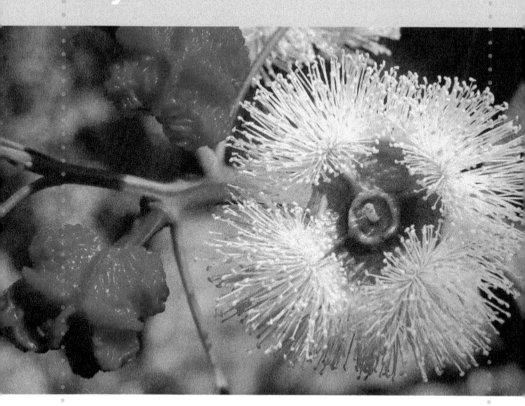

Family Myrtaceae Juss.

Botanical Name *Eucalyptus erythrocorys* F.Muell.

Common Name Illyarrie.

Noongar Name Illyarrie.

Description Illyarrie is a Eucalypt that grows to a small tree about 4 m high around Perth, but taller specimens have been sighted near Eneabba. Shorter, mallee forms have been seen in a pocket north of Geraldton. The leaves are dark green and sickle shaped. Bright yellow flowers appear from late summer to early autumn (late Buburu to early Djeran). Large, bright red, helmet-shaped fruits appear while the flowers are still present, making for a spectacular sight (ANPSA, 2016; FloraBase, 2016).

Habitat Illyarrie prefers sand in coastal and near-coastal areas (FloraBase, 2016).

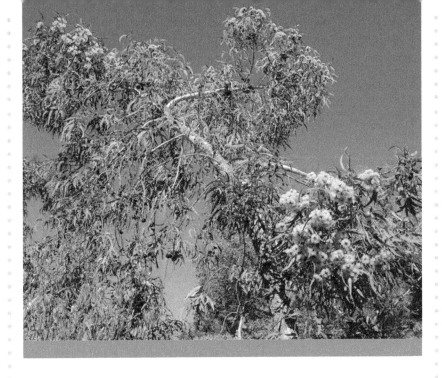

Distribution Illyarrie is native to Western Australia and is found mostly in pockets to the north and south of Geraldton (FloraBase, 2016). Because of its spectacular appearance when in flower, it is seen in many parks and gardens around Perth.

Uses For the Noongar people's use of Eucalypts, see page 24.

Active Constituents For Eucalypts' active constituents, see page 24.

Botanical Name *Acacia acuminata* Benth.

Common Names Jam Wattle, Raspberry Jam Tree, Fine Leaf Jam, Raspberry Jam, and Jam Tree.

Noongar Names Mungart, Mangart, Manjart, Munert, Munertor, Mungaitch, Mungat and Mungut (Abbott, 1983).

Description Jam Wattle grows as a tall shrub or small tree, sometimes to a height of 10 m, but is rarely found above 5 m. Its thin leaves are actually phyllodes (flattened leaf stalks) and are bright green and around 100 mm long. The prolific, bright yellow flowers appear in long clusters from July to October (late Makuru to early Kambarang) (FloraBase, 2016; World Wide Wattle, 2016).

Habitat Jam Wattle grows in a variety of soils and habitats (FloraBase, 2016).

Distribution Jam Wattle is native to the south-west of Western Australia and is seen mostly in the drier parts of the south-west from Geraldton to Esperance. It is also found around the Perth foothills (FloraBase, 2016).

Parts Used The gum and flowers.

Medicinal Uses The gum was eaten to treat diarrhoea and to aid digestion. The flowers were crushed and the vapours inhaled to relax the mind for a good night's sleep. Weak infusions of the flowers were used as washes for blisters and burns to aid healing.

Other Uses The gum mixed with water made a drink called *djilyan*.

Family Fabaceae Lindl.

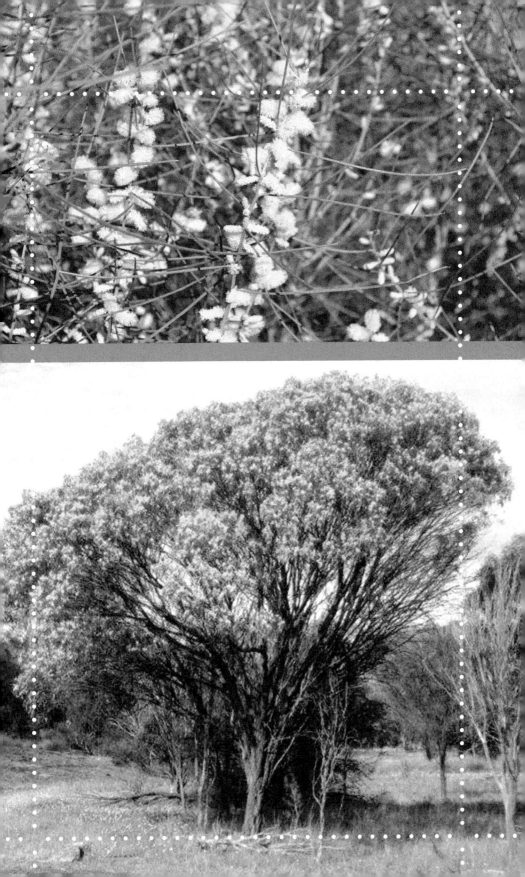

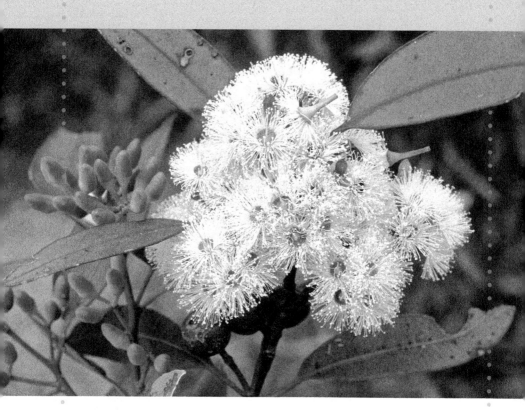

Family Myrtaceae Juss.

Botanical Name *Eucalyptus marginata* Sm.

Common Names Jarrah, and Swan River Mahogany.

Noongar Names Jarrah, Cherring, Chiaragl, Djara, Djarrail, Djarryl, Djerral, Dyerral, Gharrahel, Jarrail, Jarral, Jeerilya, Jeril, Jerrail, Jerral, Jerryl and Yarrah (City of Joondalup, 2011).

Description Jarrah is an evergreen tree that grows straight and tall to 40 m high. Its red-grey bark is rough, with vertical grooves. It sheds in long strips. The leaves are about 80–130 mm long. The tops of the leaves are dark green, while the bottoms are lighter. The white-cream or pink flowers bloom from June to January (Makuru to late Birak) (City of Mandurah, 2016; FloraBase, 2016).

Habitat Jarrah grows in a variety of soils, including grey sand, clay, sandy loam and laterite, in large forests (FloraBase, 2016).

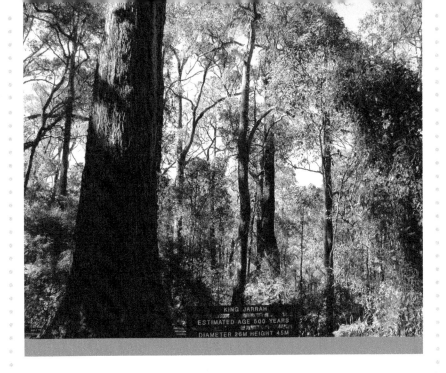

Distribution Jarrah is native to the south-west of Western Australia, growing mostly in coastal and near-coastal forests from Chittering to Bremer Bay (FloraBase, 2016).

Parts Used The leaves, gum and wood.

Medicinal Uses Jarrah gum was used as a mild anaesthetic and mixed with water and drunk to relieve diarrhoea and upset stomachs. Large pieces were sometimes used as fillings in dental cavities (City of Joondalup, 2011). For Eucalypts' other medicinal uses, see page 24.

Other Uses Jarrah timber is world famous, renowned for its toughness, durability and resistance to white ants, or termites. It is used for construction, flooring, furniture and railway sleepers. Noongar people used the bark as roofing for shelters; it was considered the best type of bark for this purpose (City of Joondalup, 2011).

Active Constituents For Eucalypts' active constituents, see page 24.

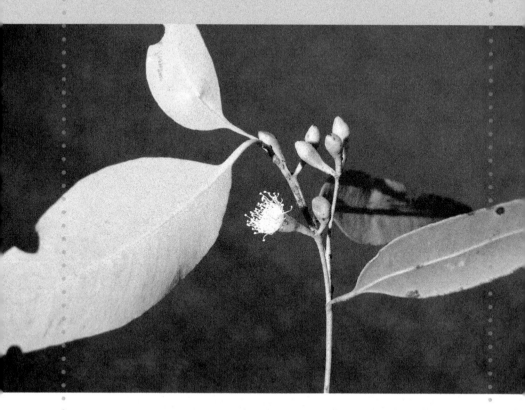

Family Myrtaceae Juss.

Botanical Name *Eucalyptus diversicolor* F.Muell.

Common Name Karri.

Noongar Names Karri, and Karril (Abbott, 1983).

Description Karri is a medium to tall forest Eucalypt that grows to around 60 m in height. It is reputed to be the tallest tree in Western Australia. It has smooth, patchy, pink and white bark. Its long leaves are dark green on the upper surface and pale green on the bottom (ANPSA, 2016). The flowers are white and appear in May (late Djeran), from September to December (late Djilba to early Birak) or from January to February (late Birak to early Bunuru) (FloraBase, 2016).

Habitat Karri prefers sand in coastal forest situations (FloraBase, 2016).

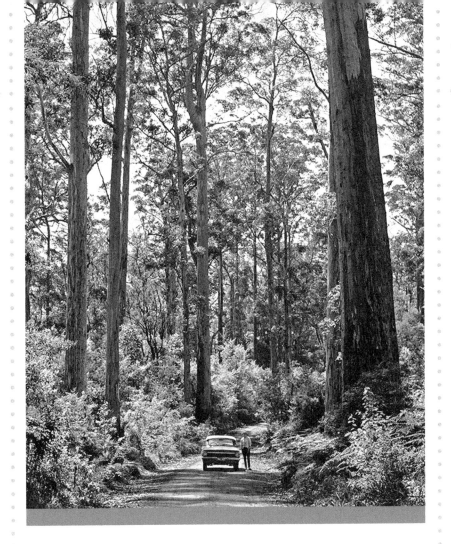

Distribution Karri is native to the higher rainfall areas of the south-west of Western Australia. It grows in forests from Busselton to Albany (FloraBase, 2016).

Parts Used The leaves, gum and wood.

Medicinal Uses For Eucalypts' medicinal uses, see page 24.

Other Uses Karri timber is prized by makers of indoor and outdoor furniture.

Active Constituents For Eucalypts' active constituents, see page 24.

Botanical Name *Trymalium odoratissimum* subsp. *trifidum* (Rye) Kellermann, Rye & K.R.Thiele.

Common Names Karri Hazel, White Hazel and Soapbush.

Noongar Names Djop Born.

Description Karri Hazel is a small shrub or tree that usually grows to around 4 m high but has been found up to 9 m high in wetter areas. It has almost oval, dark green leaves, which are pointed at the ends. Its beautiful tiny, star-shaped, white flowers appear in clusters on small branchlets in winter and spring (Makuru to Kambarang) (EKSA, n.d.).

Habitat Karri Hazel grows in sand in coastal and near-coastal areas (FloraBase, 2016).

Distribution Karri Hazel is native to the south-west of Western Australia and is found on the coastal sandplain from Perth to Bremer Bay (FloraBase, 2016).

Parts Used The leaves, twigs and flowers.

Medicinal Uses Decoctions of the plant material were added to baths to treat rheumatism and back pain, and rags soaked in the decoctions were used as poultices on swollen joints.

Other Uses Noongars placed parts of the plant into small waterholes so that animals would become groggy after drinking the affected water and were easily clubbed. The leaves produce lather similar to soap and were used to scrub hands to clean them (EKSA, n.d.).

Family Rhamnaceae Juss.

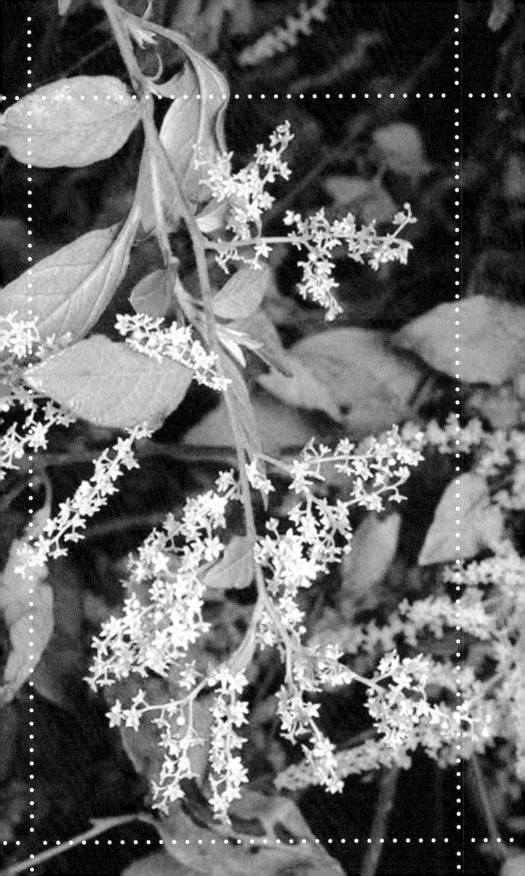

Leafless Ballart

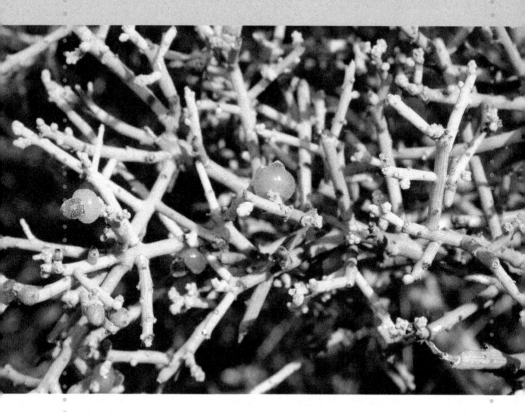

Family Santalaceae R.Br.

Botanical Name *Exocarpos aphyllus* R.Br.

Common Name Leafless Ballart.

Noongar Names Chuk, Chukk, Dtulya and Merrin (Abbott, 1983).

Other Aboriginal Name Mirnikuyan (Laverton).

Description Leafless Ballart is an erect, small tree that grows 3–5 m high. Its finely furrowed branches sometimes end in sharp points. The leaves are scale-like and are flattened against the branches (Lassak & McCarthy, 2001). The yellow-green flowers are minute. They appear from April to May (Djeran), from September to November (late Djilba to Kambarang) or in January (late Birak) depending on the conditions (FloraBase, 2016). The fruits are spherical nuts 4–5 mm in diameter (Bindon, 1996).

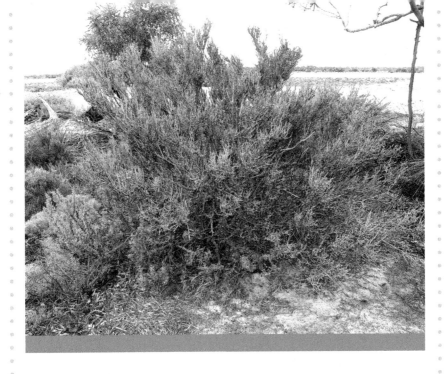

Habitat Leafless Ballart thrives in sandy loam and well-drained clay in woodland communities (Bindon, 1996).

Distribution Leafless Ballart is native to the south-west of Western Australia and is found from Shark Bay to the South Australian border (FloraBase, 2016). It is also found in inland Queensland, New South Wales and Victoria (Lassak & McCarthy, 2001).

Parts Used The stems.

Medicinal Uses Decoctions of the mashed stems were taken internally to relieve colds and applied externally to wash sores. They were also made into poultices placed on the chest to treat 'wasting diseases' (Bindon, 1996), in which muscle and fat tissue waste away – a common symptom of AIDS and cancer (Knott, 2012).

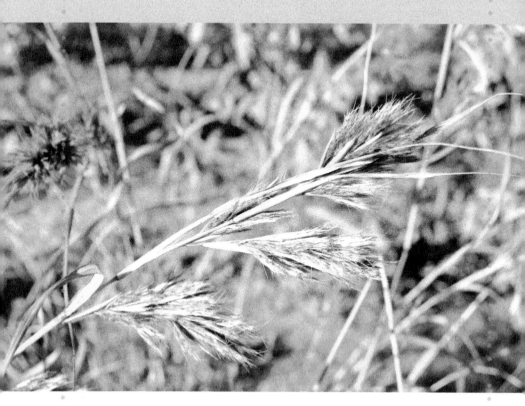

Botanical Name *Cymbopogon ambiguus* A.Camus.

Common Names Lemon Grass and Scent Grass.

Noongar Name Djerp.

Other Aboriginal Names Kalpalpi (Yuendumu) Malhanggaa Mathanguru (Yindjibarndi and Ngarluma) (Customary Medicinal Knowledgebase, 2011).

Description Lemon Grass grows in tufty clumps to around 1.8 m high. It has a lemony scent when crushed. The green flowers that appear at the tops of the grass stalks can be seen from November to December (late Kambarang to early Birak) and from January to June (late Birak to early Makuru) (FloraBase, 2016).

Habitat Lemon Grass grows on rocky hills, exposed granite and roadsides which have shallow loam or clay soil. It is also

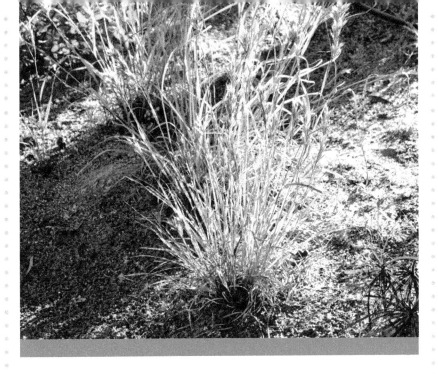

found beside creeks in stony uplands (Bowman et al., 2000; FloraBase, 2016).

Distribution Lemon Grass is found in drier areas in Western Australia. It also occurs in the Northern Territory, Queensland and New South Wales (ATRP, 2010). Good examples of this plant are found in Kings Park, Perth.

Parts Used The leaves, stems and roots. The Wajarri people used the whole plant.

Medicinal Uses Decoctions of the leaves, stems and roots were used for bathing the body to treat general illness and as washes for sores, skin rashes, cramps, earaches and sore eyes. Small amounts were drunk to relieve sore throats and diarrhoea (Olive Pink Botanic Garden, 2010). The leaves were crushed and the vapour inhaled to ease chest complaints (Pearn, 2004).

Active Constituents Grice, Rogers and Griffiths (2011) report that the essential oil contains amphene, borneol, limonene, α-pinene, α-terpineol, camphor, isoborneol, 4-terpineol, myrcene and β-ocimene. Just which of these constituents are the active ones is not known.

Mallee Riceflower

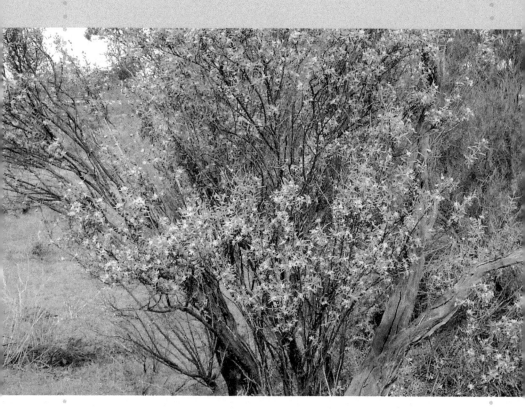

Family Thymelaeaceae Juss.

Botanical Name *Pimelea microcephala* R.Br.

Common Names Mallee Riceflower, Small-headed Riceflower, Shrub Kurrajong and Shrubby Riceflower.

Noongar Names Not known for this plant.

Other Aboriginal Names Gundagurrie (Murchison), Yackahber (St George), Willparee (Mt Lindhurst), Wondari, Wondai (Musgrave Ranges, South Australia), Wirri-pirri (Flinders Ranges) (Lassak & McCarthy, 2001).

Description Mallee Riceflower is a small shrub with many branches that grows 800 mm–2.5 m high. It has separate male and female plants. The leaves are 7–40 mm long and 1–4 mm wide. Its greenish yellow, star-shaped flowers appear in clusters in late winter or early spring (late Makuru to early Djilba). The fruits are yellow-green or red berries (Bindon, 1996).

Habitat Mallee Riceflower prefers sand and limestone in drier inland areas (Bindon, 1996; FloraBase, 2016).

Distribution Mallee Riceflower is native to the drier areas of Western Australia as well as to the rest of the Australian mainland. In the south-west, it ranges from Carnarvon and the Geraldton Sandplains through the outskirts of Noongar country to Esperance and the South Australian border (FloraBase, 2016).

Parts Used The roots, fruits and bark.

Medicinal Uses A decoction of the root was drunk by Aboriginal people for throat and chest complaints. The bark taken off the roots was effective in reducing pain when wrapped around the head or other parts of the body (Lassak and McCarthy, 2001).

Other Uses The fruits were eaten as food. The fibre of the inner bark was used for making string, fishing lines and fine mesh nets (Bindon, 1996).

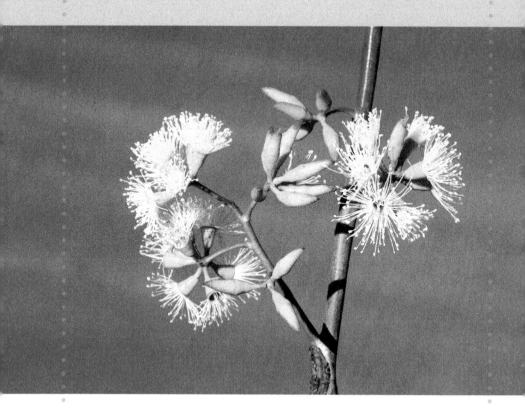

Family Myrtaceae Juss.

Botanical Name *Eucalyptus capillosa* subsp. *polyclada* Brooker & Hopper.

Common Names Mallee Wandoo, and Wheatbelt Wandoo.

Noongar Name Muruk (WNRM, 2009).

Description Mallee Wandoo is a Eucalypt growing to around 6 m in height. Its white-cream flowers appear from December to May (Birak to Djeran) (FloraBase, 2016).

Habitat Mallee Wandoo grows in a variety of soils, including gravelly sand, sandy loam and clay (FloraBase, 2016).

Distribution Mallee Wandoo is native to the drier areas in the south-west of Western Australia and is found in the Avon Wheatbelt, Mallee, Esperance Plains and as far east as Southern Cross (FloraBase, 2016).

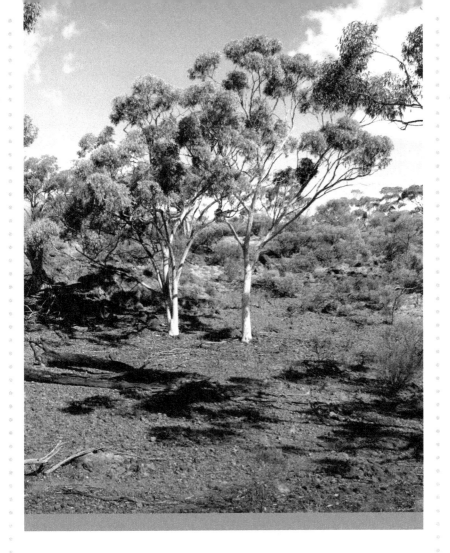

Uses For the Noongar people's use of Eucalypts, see page 24.

Active Constituents For Eucalypts' active constituents, see page 24.

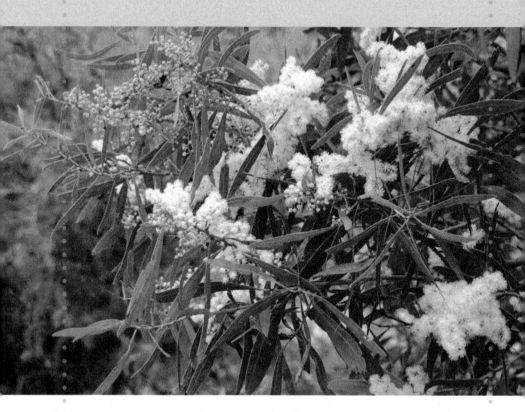

Botanical Name *Acacia microbotrya* Benth.

Common Name Manna Wattle.

Noongar Names Paadyang, Mindalong (WNRM, 2009), Badjong, Galyang, Koonert, Kunart, Kwonnat, Men and Menna (Abbott, 1983).

Description Manna Wattle is a bushy shrub or tree that grows to 7 m high. It has smooth bark, but as the tree ages the bark becomes rough at the bases of the branches. The leaves, which are actually phyllodes, are 70–140 mm long and up to 20 mm wide. The yellow-cream, globe-like flowers are spectacular and appear from March to August (late Bunuru to early Djilba) (FloraBase, 2016; World Wide Wattle, 2016).

Family Fabaceae Lindl.

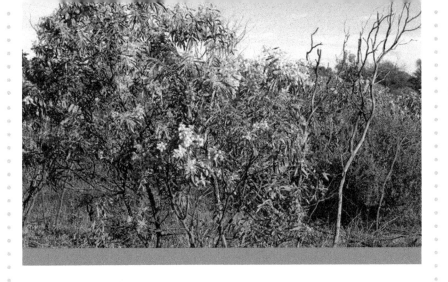

Habitat Manna Wattle grows in clay and sandy loam on granite outcrops and beside rivers and salt lakes (FloraBase, 2016).

Distribution Manna Wattle is native to the south-west of Western Australia and is widespread throughout an area from just south of Geraldton to Esperance (FloraBase, 2016).

Parts Used The inner bark, gum and seeds.

Medicinal Uses Infusions of the inner bark were used to alleviate diarrhoea. The gum was used to soothe inflamed skin (World Wide Wattle, 2013).

Other Uses The seeds and gum were eaten as food (WNRM, 2009).

Botanical Name *Scaevola spinescens* R.Br.

Common Names Maroon Bush, Cancer Bush, Prickly Fanflower and Currant Bush.

Noongar Name Murin Murin (Natural Cancer Treatment, 2015).

Description Maroon Bush is a medium-sized shrub that grows to around 2 m in height. Its leaves are long, thin and oval shaped. The fan-like, creamy-white to yellow flowers are present for most of the year. The fruits appear as small, purplish berries or currants (Crago, 2016; FloraBase, 2016).

Habitat Maroon Bush prefers sandy loam on hills in drier inland regions (Lassak & McCarthy, 2001).

Distribution Maroon Bush is found in the drier inland regions of Western Australia as well as in central Australia and New South Wales (Lassak & McCarthy, 2001). It is quite widespread in Western Australia but is found only in the drier outer areas of Noongar country (FloraBase, 2016).

Parts Used The whole plant.

Medicinal Uses Decoctions made from the whole plant were drunk to treat cancer, intestinal complaints, heart disease and urinary and kidney problems and as an immune system stimulant (Cribb & Cribb, 1983; Lassak & McCarthy, 2001). Decoctions of the stems were taken internally to treat sores and boils. The entire plant was burnt and the smoke inhaled to relieve colds.

Active Constituents According to Lassak and McCarthy (2001), furocoumarins are present in the plant, but it is not known whether they are the active medicinal constituents.

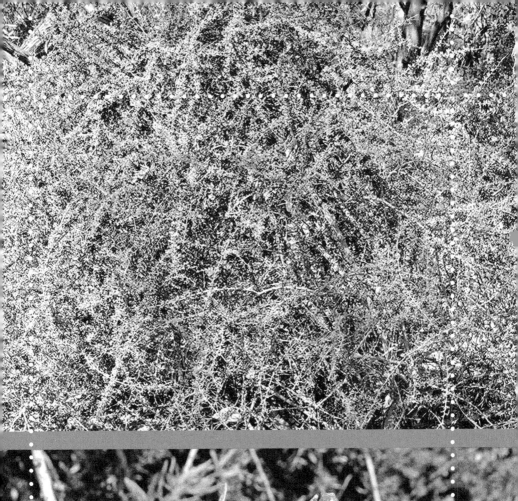

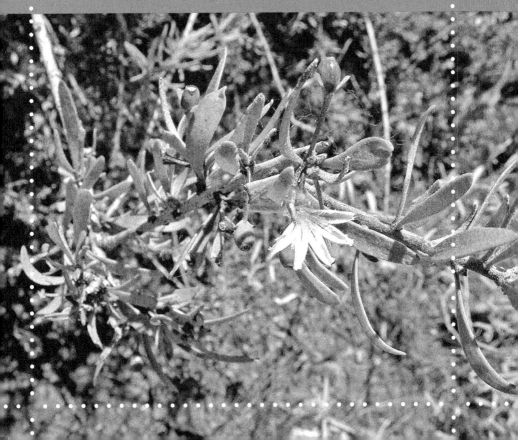

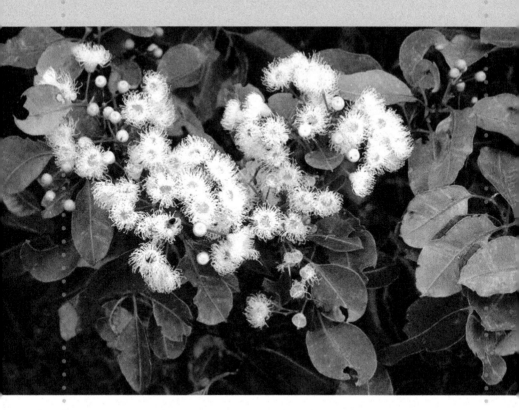

Botanical Names *Corymbia calophylla* (Lindl.) K.D.Hill & L.A.S.Johnson, formerly *Eucalyptus calophylla*.

Common Names Marri, Red Gum and Medicine Tree.

Noongar Names Marri, Mari, Marril, Marree, Mundup, Nandup, Nundup, Kurrden, Kardan, Cardau, Gardan, Grydan (City of Joondalup, 2011), Mahree, Ngora and Ngumbat (Abbott, 1983).

Description Marri is a large Eucalypt tree that can grow up to 40 m in height. Its brown bark is quite rough. The ovate leaves are pointed at the tips. The cream or pink flowers appear from December to May (Birak to Djeran). The fruits are brown and typical gumnut shapes (ANPSA, 2016).

Habitat Marri grows in a range of soils and is often found in forests amongst Jarrah and Karri (ANPSA, 2016).

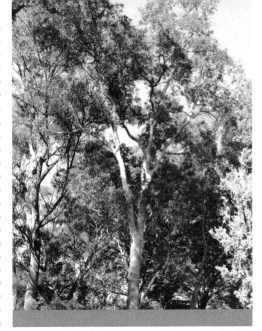

Distribution Marri is native to Western Australia and is found in coastal and some inland areas from Geraldton to Bremer Bay (FloraBase, 2016).

Parts Used The leaves, seeds, flowers and resin.

Medicinal Uses The resin, ground to a fine powder, was applied to wounds to reduce bleeding; mixed with water, it was used as medicine in small doses to treat upset stomachs and as a mouthwash and disinfectant; it was also considered a good anti-inflammatory agent and was rubbed on the skin to treat eczema (SERCUL, 2014a; UniServe Science, 2012). The resin is best if collected in the spring (late Djilba to Kambarang). The seeds were eaten as cures for diarrhoea and constipation. The leaves were crushed and the vapour inhaled to relieve headaches, sinusitis and colds. The leaves were also heated and applied to the chest to treat colds. Infusions of the flowers were taken internally as blood purifiers and to treat diabetes. The leaves were also used for smoke, as medicine to alleviate respiratory complaints.

Other Uses Smoke from the leaves was believed to be a good insect repellent. The flowers were soaked in water to make a sweet, refreshing drink called *neip*. The powdered resin was used as a tanning agent on kangaroo skins (UniServe Science, 2012).

Active Constituents For Eucalypts' active constituents, see page 24.

Mint Bush

Botanical Name *Philotheca brucei* (F.Muell.) Paul G.Wilson.

Common Name Mint Bush.

Noongar Names Not known for this plant.

Other Aboriginal Names Noolburra (Customary Medicinal Knowledgebase, 2011).

Description Mint Bush is a small shrub that grows to around 2 m high. Its thin leaves are approximately 18 mm long (Customary Medicinal Knowledgebase, 2011). The pink or white flowers appear from March to September (late Bunuru to Djilba) (FloraBase, 2016).

Habitat Mint Bush grows in a variety of soils on steep cliffs, rocky hills and outcrops (FloraBase, 2016).

Distribution Mint Bush grows only in the drier regions of southern Western Australia, from an area just north of Geraldton to just north of Perth and inland to Wiluna and Kalgoorlie (FloraBase, 2016).

Parts Used The leaves.

Medicinal Uses The leaves were crushed and placed on the head to relieve headaches and on the chest and throat to treat colds and sinus problems (Customary Medicinal Knowledgebase, 2011). Ointments made with fat and the crushed leaves were applied externally to sore glands.

Family Rutaceae Juss.

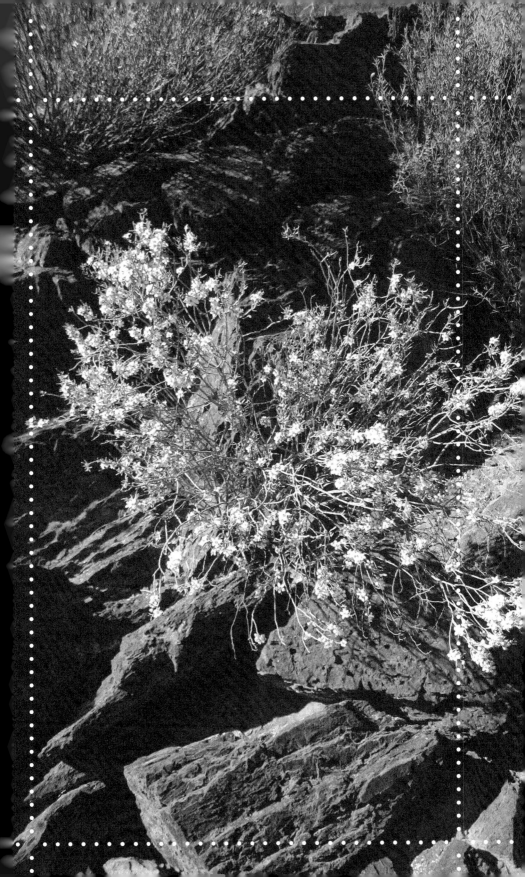

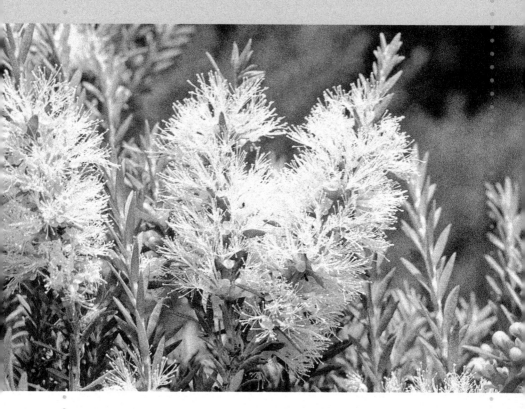

Botanical Name *Melaleuca preissiana* Schauer.

Common Names Moonah, Modong and Stout Paperbark.

Noongar Name Moonah.

Description Moonah grows as a shrub or tree 2–9 m tall. It has papery bark and short, thin, pointed leaves. Its white or cream, Bottlebrush-type flowers appear from around November to February (late Kambarang to early Bunuru) (FloraBase, 2016).

Habitat Moonah prefers sand in swampy areas on coastal sandplains (FloraBase, 2016).

Distribution Moonah is native to the south-west of Western Australia. It is found from the Geraldton Sandplains along the Swan Coastal Plain to Esperance and in the Eastern Mallee (FloraBase, 2016).

Family Myrtaceae Juss.

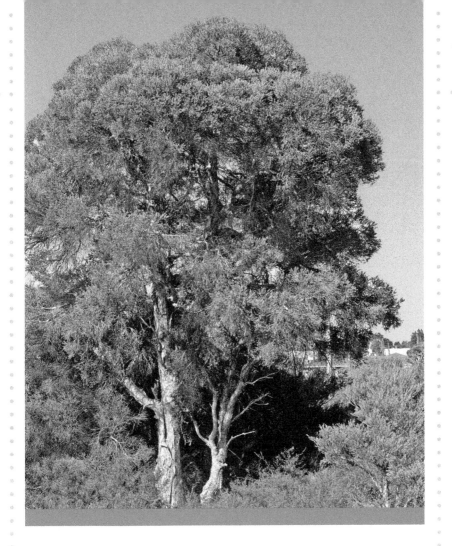

Parts Used The young leaves and bark.

Medicinal Uses The young leaves were crushed and inhaled to treat sinusitis, headaches and colds. The bark was used as bandages to bind wounds.

Other Uses The bark was used for sanitary purposes, as a natural toilet paper. It was also used to wrap food in for cooking.

Active Constituents For Melaleucas' active constituents, see page 83.

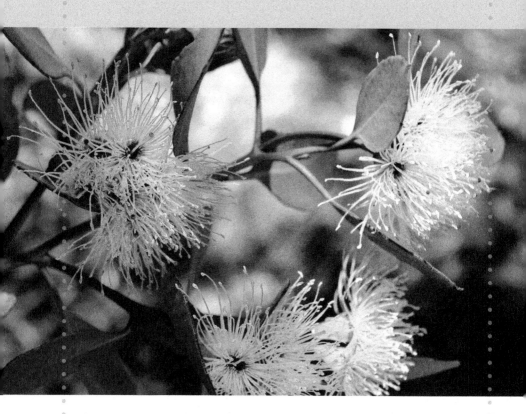

Botanical Name *Eucalyptus platypus* Hook.

Common Names Moort, Round-leaved Moort and Platypus Gum.

Noongar Names Moort and Maalok (Abbott, 1983).

Description Moort is a small to medium mallee Eucalypt that grows around 2–9 m in height. It has smooth bark, oval-shaped, light green leaves and creamy-yellow flowers that appear from September to March (late Djilba to Bunuru) (FloraBase, 2016).

Habitat Moort grows in a variety of soils, including sand, loamy clay and laterite, in coastal and near-coastal situations (FloraBase, 2016).

Distribution Moort is native to Western Australia and is found mainly along the coast between Albany and Esperance

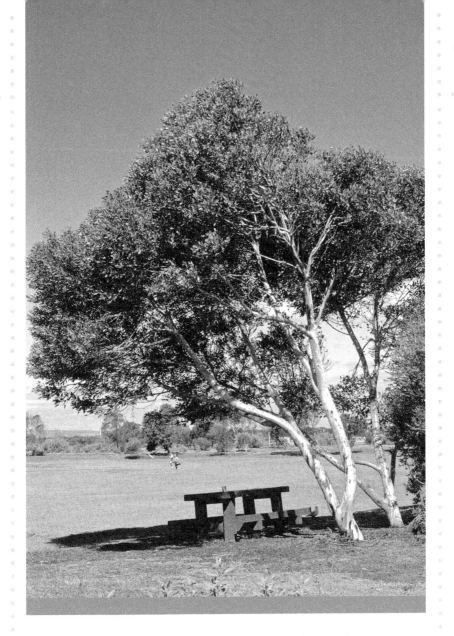

but can also be seen in the Avon Wheatbelt and the Mallee, on sandplains and in hilly and rocky country (FloraBase, 2016).

Uses For the Noongar people's use of Eucalypts, see page 24.

Active Constituents For Eucalypts' active constituents, see page 24.

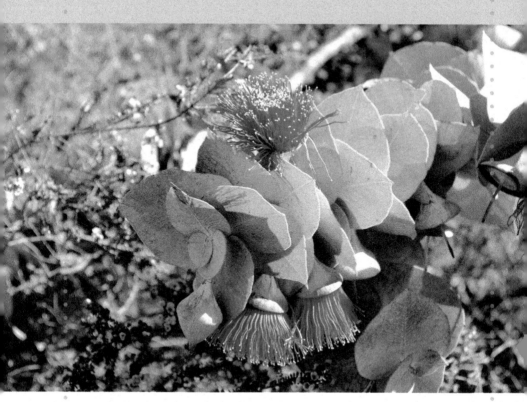

Family Myrtaceae Juss.

Botanical Name *Eucalyptus macrocarpa* Hook.

Common Name Mottlecah.

Noongar Name Mottlecar (Abbott, 1983).

Description Mottlecah is a beautiful mallee Eucalypt that grows 800 mm–5 m in height and has a spread of up to 6 m. It has silver-grey, elliptical leaves and grey bark. Its spectacular red or pink flowers appear in spring and summer (late Djilba to early Bunuru), with another flush in late autumn (late Djeran) (FloraBase, 2016). The fruits are large, bowl-shaped, light grey gumnuts (ANPSA, 2016).

Habitat Mottlecah prefers white and grey sand, sandy loam and laterite. It thrives on hill slopes, ridges and sandplains (FloraBase, 2016).

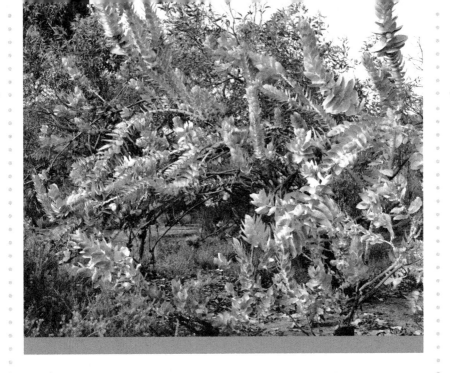

Distribution Mottlecah is native to the south-west of Western Australia. It is very prominent around the Perth area in parks and gardens but has also been recorded on the Geraldton Sandplains, in the Avon Wheatbelt, the Lesueur Sandplain and around Bruce Rock, Coorow and Quairading (FloraBase, 2016).

Uses For the Noongar people's use of Eucalypts, see page 24.

Active Constituents For Eucalypts' active constituents, see page 24.

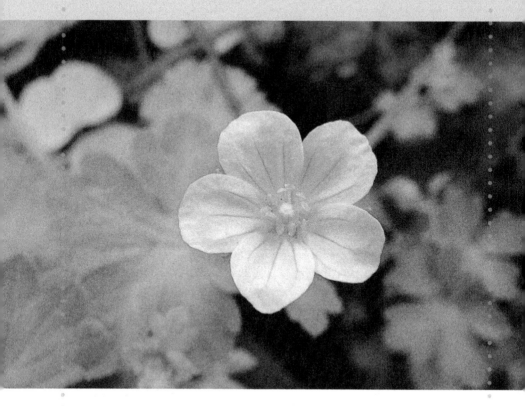

Family Geraniaceae Juss.

Botanical Name *Geranium solanderi* Carolin.

Common Names Native Geranium, Australian Cranesbill, Austral Cranesbill, Cut-leaf Cranesbill, Native Carrot and Hairy Geranium.

Noongar Names Not known for this plant.

Description Native Geranium is a spreading herb that grows to around 300 mm high. The flowers are pale pink or white, with five petals. They appear from August to December (Djilba to early Birak) (FloraBase, 2016). The plant has a large, parsnip-shaped taproot, which is edible (Greening Australia, 2016).

Habitat Native Geranium grows in a variety of soils, including sand, loam, clay, gravel and laterite over limestone, in rock crevices, on hill slopes and sand dunes, beside lakes and in coastal areas (FloraBase, 2016).

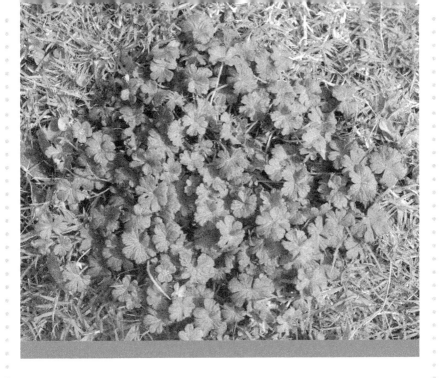

Distribution Native Geranium is native to the south-west of Western Australia and is found growing from around Cervantes north of Perth to Albany. There are also patches growing around Esperance. Native Geranium is also found in the Eastern States from south-west Queensland around to the south-east of South Australia (Atlas of Living Australia, 2016).

Parts Used The roots.

Medicinal Uses The older (red) tuberous roots were pounded and then cooked and eaten to treat diarrhoea (BACC, 2016).

Native Plantain

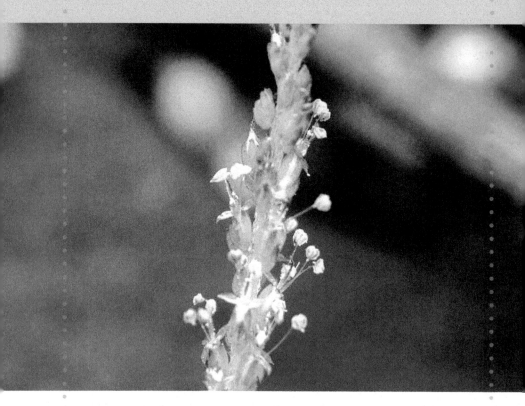

Family Plantaginaceae Juss.

Botanical Name *Plantago debilis* R.Br.

Common Names Native Plantain, and Shade Plantain.

Noongar Names Not known for this plant.

Description Native Plantain is a ground-hugging herb with a slender tap root. Its dark green, hairy leaves, around 60 mm long and with toothed edges, rise from the base of the plant (NSWFO, 2016). The small, white flowers appear on one or two stalks from August to December (Djilba to early Birak) (FloraBase, 2016).

Habitat Native Plantain grows in sand in moist areas of open forest and grassland (FloraBase, 2016).

Distribution Native Plantain is found all over southern Australia, including Tasmania (NSWFO, 2016). In Western Australia, it is found throughout the south-west from Jurien

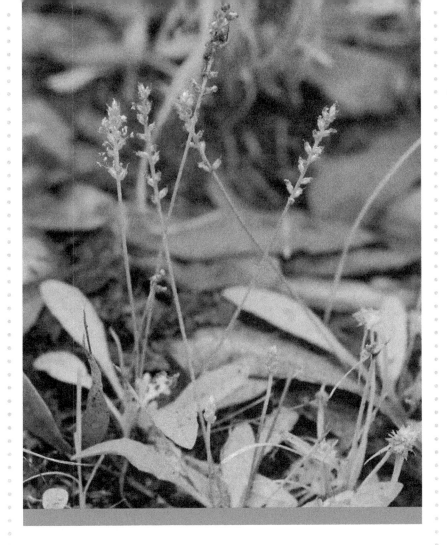

Bay to Esperance and inland beyond Kalgoorlie (FloraBase, 2016).

Parts Used The leaves.

Medicinal Uses When warmed and crushed, the leaves yield a sap that was used to draw swelling from sprains and as a poultice on sores, such as ulcers, boils and carbuncles (NMNR, 2013).

Old Man Saltbush

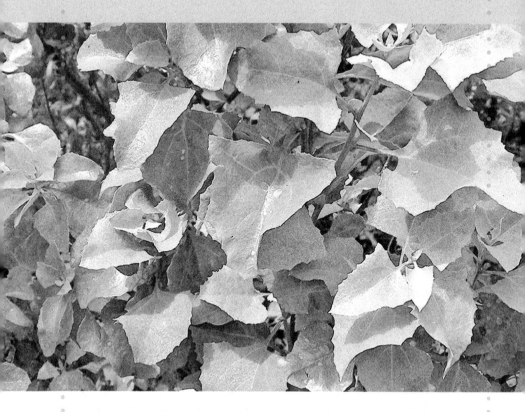

Family Chenopodiaceae Vent.

Botanical Name *Atriplex nummularia* Lindl.

Common Names Old Man Saltbush, Bluegreen Saltbush, Cabbage Saltbush and Giant Saltbush.

Noongar Names Purngep, Pining (Esperance) and Binga.

Description Old Man Saltbush is a shrub that grows to around 3 m high. It can have a spread of up to 4 m. The plant has oval, scaly, silver-grey leaves that can have toothed edges. The small, pale red, star-shaped flowers that have five petals appear at different time throughout the year depending on the conditions. The plant has male and female flowers (Department of Primary Industry, 2010; Lassak & McCarthy, 2001).

Habitat Old Man Saltbush prefers clay and sand in drier regions (FloraBase, 2016; Lassak & McCarthy, 2001).

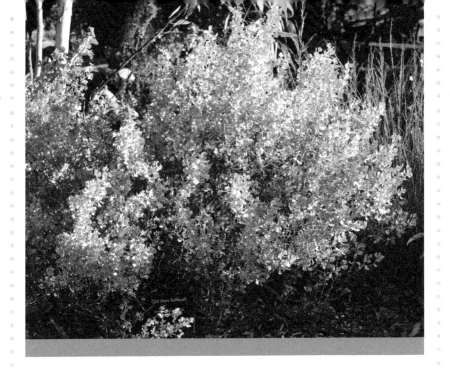

Distribution Old Man Saltbush is found from the drier regions of the south-west of Western Australia to South Australia, Victoria, New South Wales and south-western Queensland (FloraBase, 2016; Lassak & McCarthy, 2001). Good examples of this plant can be seen in Kings Park, Perth.

Parts Used The leaves and roots.

Medicinal Uses Decoctions of the leaves were used externally as skin cleansers and to bathe skin sores, burns and wounds. Early settlers were reported to have used Old Man Saltbush to treat scurvy and blood disorders (Lassak and McCarthy, 2001).

Other Uses Grubs found in the root systems were eaten, raw or roasted. A leaf was placed under the tongue to prevent dehydration.

Pale Turpentine Bush

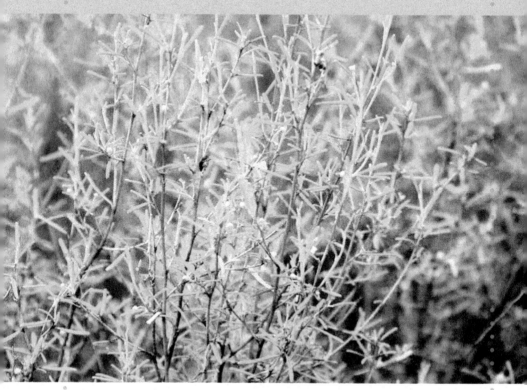

Botanical Name *Beyeria lechenaultii* (DC.) Baill.

Common Names Pale Turpentine Bush and Felted Wallaby Bush.

Noongar Names Not known for this plant.

Description Pale Turpentine Bush grows as a small bush or shrub to around 1.5 m tall. The narrow leaves appear white with hairy undersides (Lassak and McCarthy, 2001). The yellow-green flowers appear from August to December (Djilba to early Birak) (FloraBase, 2016).

Habitat Pale Turpentine Bush grows in a variety of soils, including sand, sandy loam and clay. It is found on sand dunes, rocky outcrops and flats and beside wetlands (FloraBase, 2016).

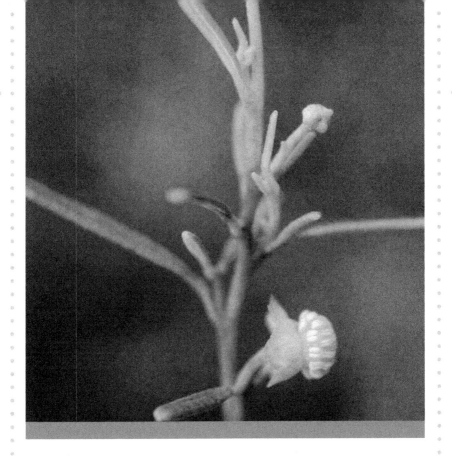

Distribution Pale Turpentine Bush grows in the more arid southern regions of Western Australia, South Australia, New South Wales, Victoria and Tasmania (Atlas of Living Australia, 2016; Lassak & McCarthy, 2001). In the south-west of Western Australia, it grows in drier regions from just north of Perth to beyond Esperance (FloraBase, 2016).

Parts Used The leaves.

Medicinal Uses Decoctions of the crushed leaves were taken internally to treat tuberculosis and fevers (Cribb & Cribb, 1983; Lassak & McCarthy, 2001).

Active Constituents Lassak and McCarthy (2001) report that the resin coating on the stems contains triterpenoid alcohols. However, whether these alcohols are responsible for the plant's medicinal effects is not known.

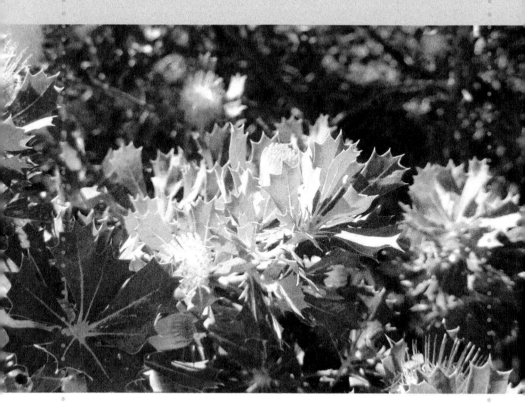

Botanical Names *Banksia sessilis* (Knight) A.R.Mast & K.R.Thiele, formerly *Dryandra sessilis*.

Common Name Parrot Bush.

Noongar Names Pulgart (City of Joondalup, 2011) and Budjan (Abbott, 1983).

Description Parrot Bush grows as a shrub or small tree up to 5 m in height. It has oval, dark green leaves with spiky edges. Its small, dome-shaped, yellow, spiky flowers appear from April to November (Djeran to Kambarang) (FloraBase, 2016).

Habitat Parrot Bush grows in a variety of soils, including sand over limestone and laterite (FloraBase, 2016).

Distribution Parrot Bush is native to Western Australia and is widespread throughout the south-west of the state on

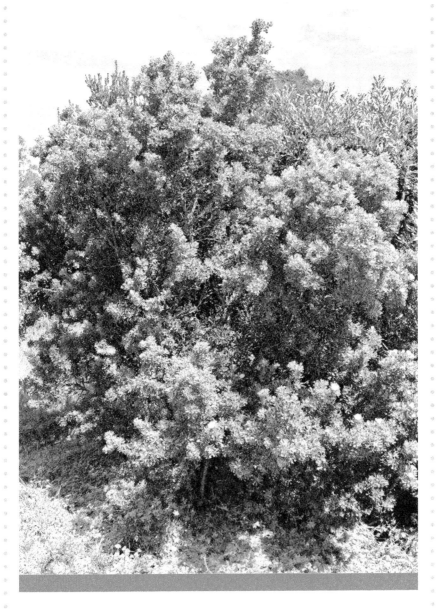

coastal sandplains from just north of Perth to Bremer Bay. It is also found in the Avon Wheatbelt (FloraBase, 2016).

Uses For the Noongar people's use of Banksias, see page 16.

Pukati

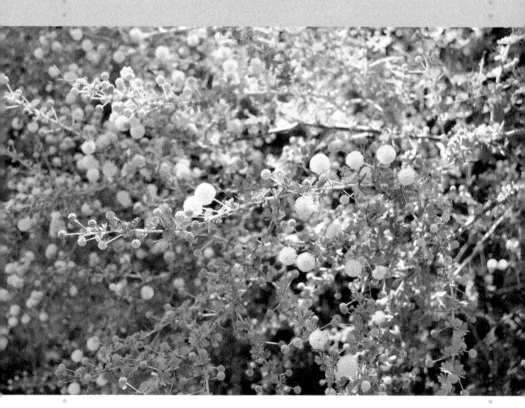

Family Fabaceae Lindl.

Botanical Name *Acacia beauverdiana* Ewart & Sharman.

Common Name Pukati.

Noongar Name Pukkati (Lassak & McCarthy, 2001).

Description Pukati is a Wattle that grows as a shrub or small tree to around 6 m in height. Its leaves, which are actually phyllodes, are long and thin and grow to around 100 mm in length (Lassak & McCarthy, 2001). Its globular, yellow flowers appear from July to October (late Makuru to early Kambarang) (FloraBase, 2016).

Habitat Pukati grows in coarse sand and sandy gravel in drier areas (Lassak and McCarthy, 2001).

Distribution Pukati is native to the semi-arid regions of the south-west of Western Australia and is seen frequently

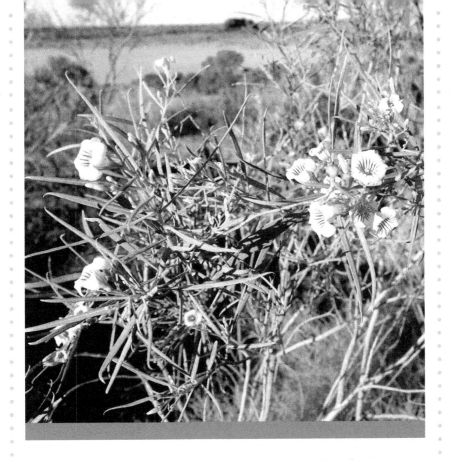

in the Mallee (Lassak and McCarthy, 2001) and as far east as Coolgardie and Esperance (Florabase, 2016).

Part Used The branches.

Medicinal Uses The small top branches were burnt and their ash mixed with equal parts of the Native Tobacco, or Pituri (*Duboisia hopwoodii*), as pictured above and chewed as a narcotic to relieve toothaches and other intense pains (Lassak & McCarthy, 2001; Taste Australia, 2016).

Active Constituents An alkaline substance that is present in the ash of the burnt branches is believed to be the active constituent of Pukati. It is reported to release the alkaloids from the Native Tobacco thus increasing the narcotic effect (Lassak & McCarthy, 2001).

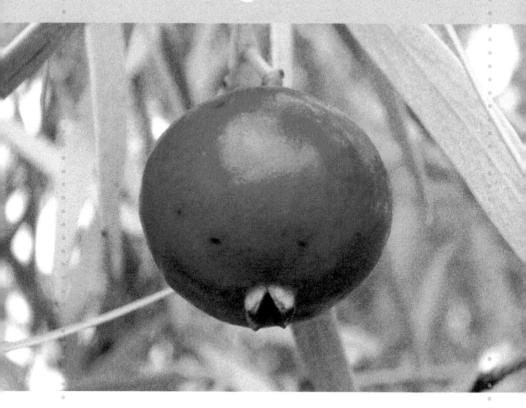

Botanical Name *Santalum acuminatum* (R.Br.) A.DC.

Common Names Quandong, Sandalwood, Desert Quandong, Sweet Quandong and Native Peach.

Noongar Names Dumbari, Jawirli, Walku, Wanga, Wayanu, Wongil (Coppin, 2008), Candang, Wong, Wonyill and Wolgol (Abbott, 1983; Bindon & Chadwick, 2011).

Other Aboriginal Names Kelango, Mangarta, Mangirta and Gutchu.

Description Quandong is one of the many types of Sandalwoods. It is semi-parasitic and grows as a large shrub or small tree to 7 m in height. It has long, thin, greyish-green leaves and rough bark. The small, white flowers occur in clusters from January to April (late Birak to early Djeran), from July to September (late Makuru to Djilba) or from November

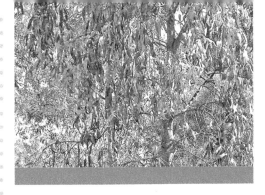

to December (late Kambarang to early Birak). After it flowers, fleshy fruits appear, which are bright red when they ripen. The round seeds inside the fruits have hard, woody shells (ANPSA, 2016).

Habitat Quandong prefers sand and clayey loam and is found in a wide range of habitats, including sandplains, around granite outcrops and near watercourses (FloraBase, 2016).

Distribution Quandong grows in many parts of Australia, including coastal south-west Western Australia, the southern Northern Territory, most of South Australia, New South Wales and south-western Queensland (ANBG, 2002). In Western Australia, it is found throughout the south-west from Shark Bay to Esperance and inland beyond Kalgoorlie (FloraBase, 2016).

Parts Used The seeds, fruits and leaves.

Medicinal Uses The seed kernels, ground and mixed with animal fat, were used as a liniment to relieve sore muscles. The leaves were pounded to a paste and applied to sores and boils and were used to treat gonorrhoea (Lassak & McCarthy, 2001). Infusions of the leaves were used as treatment for diabetes.

Other Uses Traditionally, Aboriginal people ate the raw flesh of the fruits or dried and stored it for later use. It is high in vitamin C and various minerals, and low in sugar (Australian Seed, 2016). A paste made from the ground seeds was used as a skin moisturiser.

Active Constituents The nuts are rich in a fixed oil. The active constituents of the leaves are not known (Lassak & McCarthy, 2001).

Red-eyed Wattle

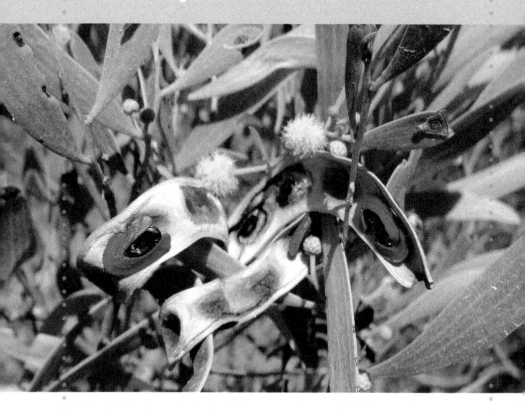

Family Fabaceae Lindl.

Botanical Name *Acacia cyclops* G.Don.

Common Names Red-eyed Wattle, Cyclops Wattle, One-eyed Wattle, Red-eye, Red Wreath Acacia and Western Coastal Wattle.

Noongar Names Munyuret, Woolya Wah and Wilyawa (City of Joondalup, 2011).

Description Red-eyed Wattle usually grows as a dense shrub but can form a small tree up to 4 m high. Its thick, green, leathery leaves, which are actually phyllodes, can reach up to 90 mm in length. The yellow, globe-shaped flowers appear from September to December (late Djilba to early Birak) or from January to May (late Birak to Djeran) depending on the area. The name 'Cyclops Wattle' comes from the one-eyed appearance of the seed pods, which are twisted and around 150 mm long (FloraBase, 2016; World Wide Wattle, 2016).

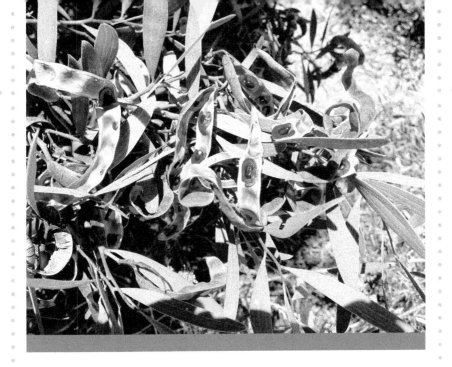

Habitat Red-eyed Wattle prefers white and grey sand. Its main habitats are coastal sand dunes and the tops of limestone cliffs (FloraBase, 2016).

Distribution Red-eyed Wattle is a coastal species, occurring from Jurien Bay to the south coast and eastwards into South Australia and Kangaroo Island (FloraBase, 2016; World Wide Wattle, 2016).

Parts Used The leaves, seeds and stems.

Medicinal Uses The juice of the leaves, extracted by crushing them, was used for relieving eczema (City of Joondalup, 2011; YMNAI, 2008).

Other Uses The seeds were ground into flour and baked into damper (City of Joondalup, 2011; YMNAI, 2008), and their juice was used as insect repellent and sunscreen. According to SERCUL (2014b), the stems contain gum and the larvae of grubs (a nutritious food), both of which were eaten.

Red-flowering Gum

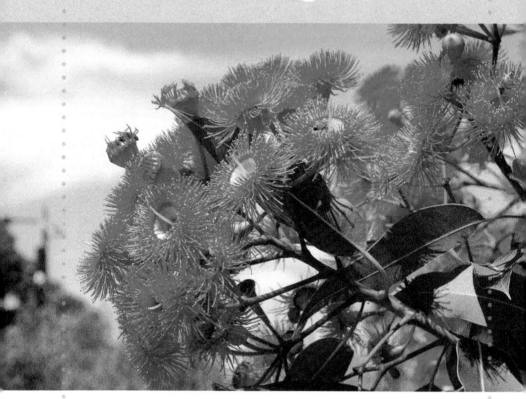

Family Myrtaceae Juss.

Botanical Name *Corymbia ficifolia* (F.Muell.) K.D.Hill & L.A.S.Johnson.

Common Name Red-flowering Gum.

Noongar Names Boorn and Yorgam.

Description Red-flowering Gum is a Eucalypt that grows from 2–10 m high depending on the conditions. It has green, ovate leaves with pointy ends, and its bark is rough and grooved. The red-orange flowers for which it is noted appear from December to May (Birak to Djeran) (FloraBase, 2016).

Habitat Red-flowering Gum is found in sandy loam and gravel on hill slopes (FloraBase, 2016).

Distribution Red-flowering Gum is native to a part of the south-west of Western Australia around Denmark and Albany (FloraBase, 2016). However, because of its beautiful

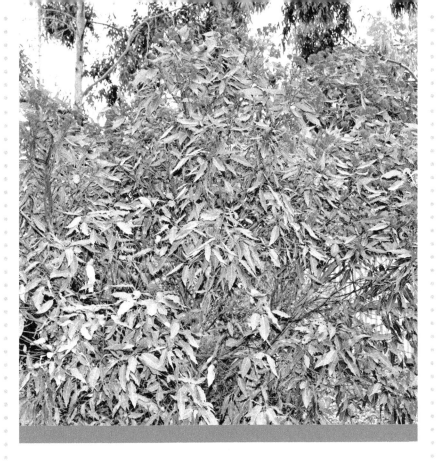

appearance, it is a feature of many parks and gardens around Perth and other towns in the south-west.

Uses For the Noongar people's use of Eucalypts, see page 24.

Active Constituents For Eucalypts' active constituents, see page 24.

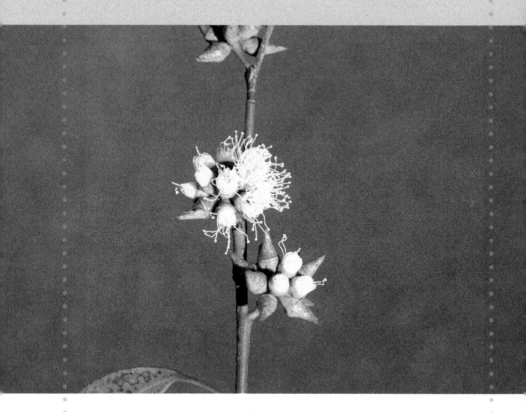

Botanical Name *Eucalyptus decipiens* Endl.

Common Names Red Heart Gum and Redheart Moit.

Noongar Names Moit (Bennett, 1991).

Description Red Heart Gum is a Eucalypt that grows as a mallee or tree up to 15 m high. Its bark is rough and flaky or ribbony. The dull grey-green leaves are almost oval and are tapered at the bases. The white flowers appear from August to January (Djilba to Birak). The fruits (gumnuts) are hemispherical (Eucalink, 2004; FloraBase, 2016).

Habitat Red Heart Gum grows in a variety of soils including sand, clay and loams. Its habitats include sandplains, slopes and swampy areas (FloraBase, 2016).

Distribution Red Heart Gum is native to the south-west of Western Australia and is found on sandplains from Geraldton

Family **Myrtaceae Juss.**

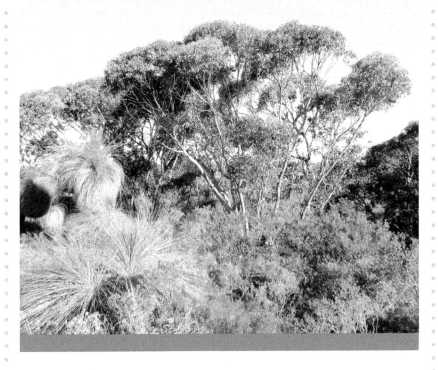

to Esperance and in the Avon Wheatbelt (FloraBase, 2016).

Uses For the Noongar people's use of Eucalypts,
see page 24.

Active Constituents For Eucalypts' active constituents,
see page 24.

Red Morrel

Botanical Name *Eucalyptus longicornis* (F.Muell.) Maiden.

Common Name Red Morrel.

Noongar Names Morryl, Poot and Put (Abbott, 1983).

Description Red Morrel is a medium to tall Eucalypt tree or mallee that grows up to 30 m in height. It has rough, grey, stringy bark up to the branches, with smooth, grey bark on the branches. The leaves are oval shaped and are grey-green in colour. The white or creamy-yellow flowers appear from November to March (late Kambarang to Bunuru). The fruits are globe-like capsules (EucaLink, 2004; FloraBase, 2016).

Habitat Red Morrel prefers loam and clayey loam on flat country (FloraBase, 2016).

Distribution Red Morrel is native to the south-west of

Family **Myrtaceae Juss.**

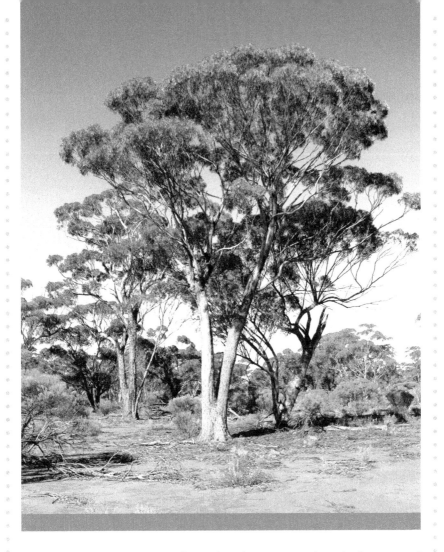

Western Australia and is found in the Avon Wheatbelt, around Wickepin, and as far east as Norseman and Coolgardie (Florabank, 2016; FloraBase, 2016).

Uses For the Noongar people's use of Eucalypts, see page 24.

Active Constituents For Eucalypts' active constituents, see page 24.

Botanical Name *Banksia occidentalis* R.Br.

Common Names Red Swamp Banksia and Waterbush.

Noongar Names Mo, Yundill (Abbott, 1983), Mangatj, and Pia.

Description Red Swamp Banksia grows as a shrub or small tree up to 7 m high. It has smooth, grey-brown bark. Its leaves are long and thin and can be up to 130 mm in length. The flowers appear mainly in summer and autumn (Birak to Djeran) and are bright red, cylindrical spikes, although pink and yellow flowers have been seen near Denmark, on the south coast (ANPSA, 2016).

Habitat Red Swamp Banksia prefers sandy soils around sand dunes and swampy areas (FloraBase, 2016).

Distribution Red Swamp Banksia is native to the south-west of Western Australia. It occurs along the south coast from Busselton to Esperance (FloraBase, 2016).

Uses For the Noongar people's use of Banksias, see page 16.

Family Proteaceae Juss.

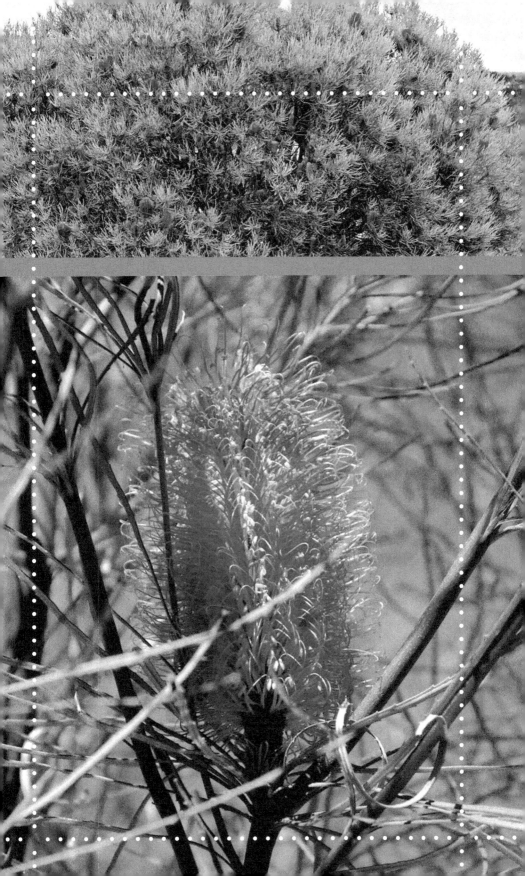

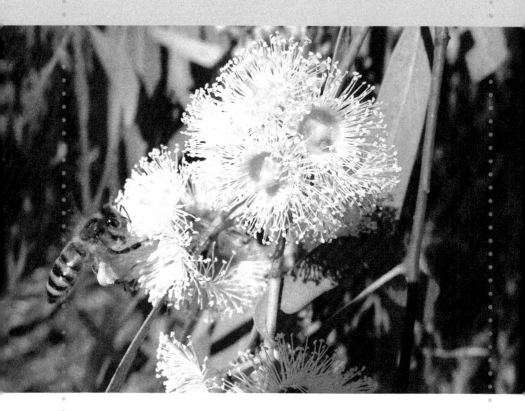

Botanical Name *Eucalyptus camaldulensis* Dehnh.

Common Names River Red Gum and Murray Red Gum.

Noongar Names Gyrdan and Kardan (Bindon & Chadwick, 2011).

Other Aboriginal Names Biall, Yarrah, Moolerr Polak (Lassak & McCarthy, 2001).

Description River Red Gum is a medium-sized Eucalypt known to reach up to 40 m in height. The tree usually branches just above the ground. The bark is rough near the bottom of the tree and has a smooth, white or greyish coloured bark further up the trunks. The blue-grey leaves are lance-shaped and are around 250 mm long. The white flowers can appear at any time from July to February (late

Family Myrtaceae Juss.

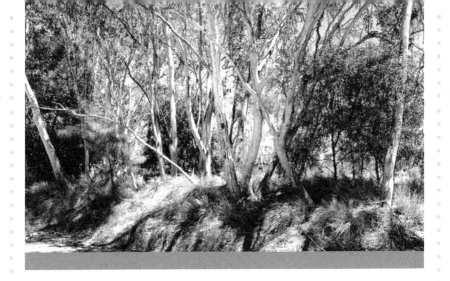

Makuru to early Bunuru). Small seed capsules appear after the tree finishes flowering (ANPSA, 2016; FloraBase, 2016).

Habitat River Red Gum grows in a variety of soils, including grey, heavy clay and red sand. It is common and widespread beside rivers and creeks (CSIRO, 2004; FloraBase, 2016).

Distribution River Red Gum is found throughout much of mainland Australia (CSIRO, 2004). It occurs in central and northern parts of Western Australia but is more common from just north of Geraldton to Bunbury (FloraBase, 2016).

Parts Used The leaves, gum, wood, seeds and bark.

Medicinal Uses Washes made from the bark, by soaking the bark in water, were used externally to treat sores and wounds and to stop bleeding (Lassak & McCarthy, 2001). For Eucalypts' other medicinal uses, see page 24.

Other Uses The timber was used for making canoes, shields, *coolamons* (carrying dishes), boomerangs, digging sticks and shelters (Monash University, 2010). The raw seeds were eaten.

Active Constituents For Eucalypts' active constituents, see page 24.

Rock Isotome

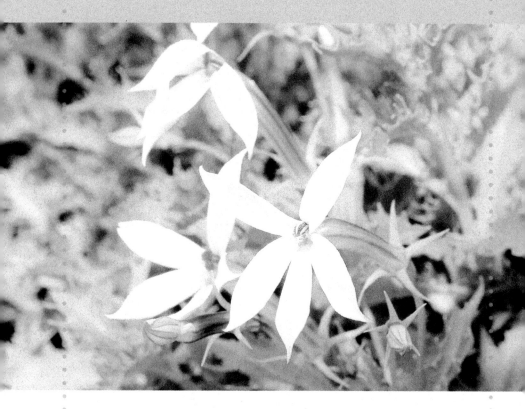

Botanical Names *Isotoma petraea* F.Muell., also known as *Laurentia petraea* (F.Muell.) E.Wimm.

Common Names Rock Isotome and Wild Tobacco.

Noongar Names Not known for this plant.

Other Aboriginal Names Minekalpa, Tundi-wari, Pulbawari, Pitherr, Anterlp, Irranerratye, Ntereympe, Mara-kanyala, Tjuntiwari, Wanngati, Multu and Yarrampa (Customary Medicinal Knowledgebase, 2011).

Description Rock Isotome is a small plant that grows up to 300 mm tall. The leaves are oblong and sharply toothed. The pale blue or blue-purple flowers have five petals and appear from February to November (Bunuru to Kambarang). The fruits are egg shaped and around 20 mm long (Bindon, 1996; FloraBase, 2016).

Family Campanulaceae Juss.

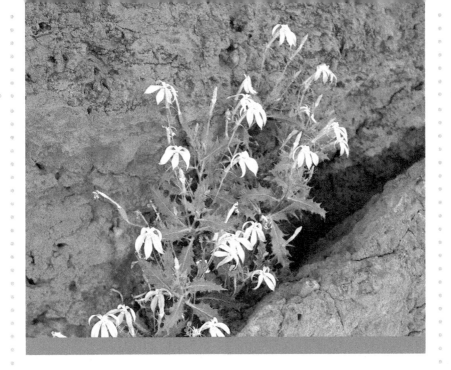

Habitat Rock Isotome thrives in shallow soil in rocky environments and caves (FloraBase, 2016; Lassak & McCarthy, 2001).

Distribution Rock Isotome is native to Western Australia and is found in the drier areas of the state. In the south-west, it appears to be confined to the drier, outer reaches of Noongar country from Geraldton to Esperance (FloraBase, 2016). It is also found in the drier areas of all mainland Australia (Lassak & McCarthy, 2001).

Parts Used The whole plant.

Medicinal Uses The plant was chewed for its narcotic and stimulant effects. In some parts of Australia, the dried and powdered plant mixed with equal parts of Mulga Tree (*Acacia aneura*) ash was ingested as a painkiller and to treat colds. Lassak and McCarthy (2001) believe that the ash may have served to release the alkaloids from the plant material.

Active Constituents Lassak and McCarthy (2001) believe a nicotine-like alkaloid that is present in the leaves could be the active constituent of Rock Isotome.

Botanical Name *Callitris preissii* Miq.

Common Names Rottnest Island Pine and Betadine Tree.

Noongar Name Marro (Abbott, 1983).

Description Rottnest Island Pine is a medium-sized tree that grows to around 10 m tall. It can have a spread of up to 9 m. Its small, brown-yellow-orange flowers appear from October to January (Kambarang to Birak) (FloraBase, 2016). The tree develops globe-shaped, woody cones that are about 20 mm wide. They rely on decay to release their seeds (Florabank, 2016).

Habitat Rottnest Island Pine grows in a variety of soils, including sand, loam and laterite in a range of habitats including sandplains, hill slopes and around salt lakes (FloraBase, 2016).

Distribution This species is native to the Swan Coastal Plain around Perth and to Rottnest and Garden islands in the south-west of Western Australia (Florabank, 2016). It is also found in large numbers between Kalgoorlie and Esperance and has been seen near Denmark and Albany (FloraBase, 2016).

Parts Used The leaves, stems, bark and nuts.

Medicinal Uses The leaves, bark and stems were used as smoke medicine for respiratory problems. Infusions of the herb were used as chest rubs to relieve coughs and colds, were rubbed around the back of the neck and the nasal area to treat sinusitis and were used as washes for burns and insect bites. Poultices made from the bark were placed on the chest for treatment of congestion. The nuts were pounded to extract the liquid inside, which was squeezed onto the skin to relieve sores, rashes and other skin irritations.

Family Cupressaceae Gray.

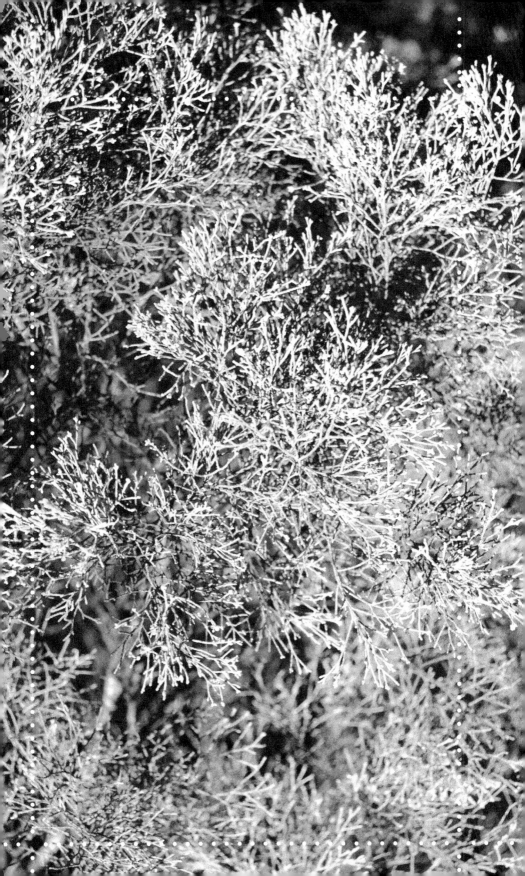

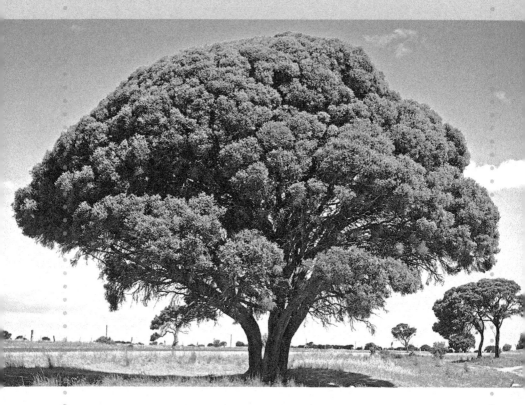

Botanical Name *Melaleuca lanceolata* Otto.

Common Names Rottnest Island Teatree and Black Paperbark.

Noongar Names Moonah (Bennett, 1991).

Description Rottnest Island Teatree grows as a large shrub or small tree to 10 m in height. It has rough bark. Its long, narrow elliptical leaves grow to around 15 mm in length. The white-cream, Bottlebrush-type flowers are seen up to 40 mm long. They can appear at any time from January to September (late Birak to Djilba) but are seen mainly in summer (Birak to early Bunuru) (Florabank, 2016; FloraBase, 2016).

Habitat Rottnest Island Teatree grows in a variety of soils, including sand, clay and loam. It is found in a range of

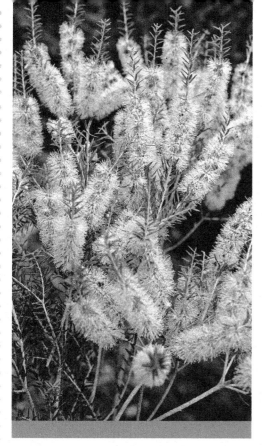

habitats including limestone ridges, sand dunes and around salt lakes. (FloraBase, 2016).

Distribution Rottnest Island Teatree, as well as being native to and a feature of Rottnest Island, grows throughout the south-west of Western Australia (FloraBase, 2016). It is also found in the southern reaches of South Australia, Victoria, New South Wales and Queensland (NSWFO, 2016).

Parts Used The leaves and stems.

Medicinal Uses The leaves were crushed and the vapour inhaled to relieve congestion (Glasby, 2016). The leaves and stems were also crushed, heated and applied to the body as poultices for aches and pains.

Active Constituents For Melaleucas' active constituents, see page 83.

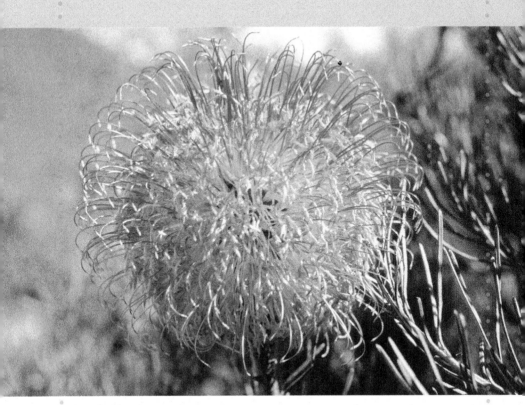

Family Proteaceae Juss.

Botanical Name *Banksia sphaerocarpa* R.Br.

Common Names Round-fruit Banksia and Fox Banksia.

Noongar Name Nugoo.

Description Round-fruit Banksia is a shrub that grows to around 2 m high. It has very narrow, green leaves and brownish orange, almost spherical flowers, which appear at any time from January to October (late Birak to early Kambarang) (ANPSA, 2016; FloraBase, 2016).

Habitat Round-fruit Banksia prefers sand in scrubland and woodland (ANPSA, 2016; FloraBase, 2016).

Distribution Round-fruit Banksia is native to the south-west of Western Australia and is widely distributed from Geraldton to the Esperance Plains (FloraBase, 2016).

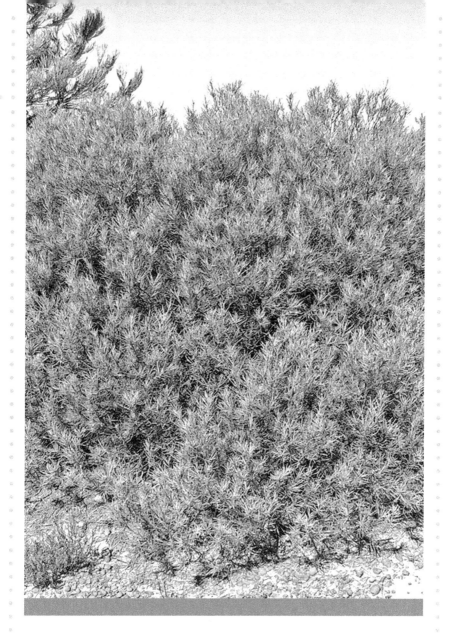

Uses For the Noongar people's use of Banksias, see page 16.

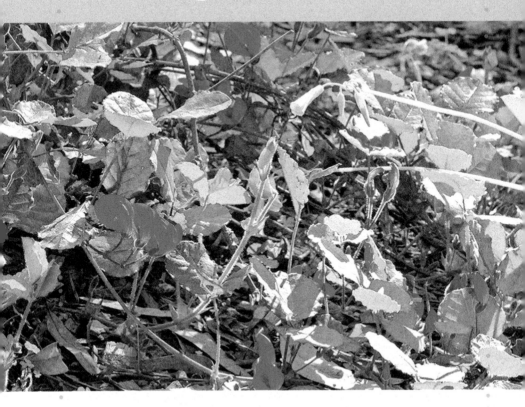

Family Fabaceae.

Botanical Name *Kennedia prostrata* R.Br.

Common Names Running Postman and Scarlet Runner.

Noongar Name Wollung.

Description Running Postman grows as a prostrate ground cover with a spread of around 2.5 m. Its grey-green leaves have three segments and wavy, yellow edges. The pea-shaped, bright red flowers appear from April to November (Djeran to late Kambarang). Flat seed pods about 50 mm long are present when flowering finishes (ANPSA, 2016). The plant has the ability to die back in dry conditions and spring to life again when it rains.

Habitat Running Postman prefers moist sand and gravel (FloraBase, 2016). Its habitats include forests, woodlands and heathy grasslands (ANPSA (2016).

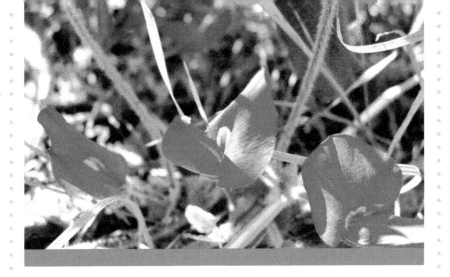

Distribution Running Postman grows throughout southern Australia, from Geraldton to Esperance in the south-west of Western Australia to the north-east of New South Wales (ANPSA, 2016).

Parts Used The flowers, stems and leaves.

Medicinal Uses The nectar from the flowers was used to soothe sore throats.

Other Uses The leaves were used to make a tea-like, refreshing drink. The stems were made into twine for tying things together.

Salmon Gum

Botanical Name *Eucalyptus salmonophloia* F.Muell.

Common Name Salmon Gum.

Noongar Names Warak, Woonert (WNRM, 2009), Worrick, Wurukk (Bindon & Chadwick, 2011) and Weerluk (Abbott, 1983).

Description Salmon Gum is a Eucalypt that grows to a height of 30 m. As its common name suggests, it has salmon-coloured, smooth bark, which appears grey in winter. The glossy, grey-green leaves are long, lance shaped and tapered at the ends (FPCWA, 2016). The white-cream flowers appear from August to December (Djilba to early Birak) (FloraBase, 2016).

Habitat Salmon Gum is found in a variety of soils, sand and clayey loam on both sandplains and in hilly areas. (FloraBase, 2016).

Distribution Salmon Gum is native to the south-west of Western Australia and is found inland from the Geraldton Sandplains to the Esperance Plains and as far east as the Eastern Mallee beyond Kalgoorlie (FloraBase, 2016).

Uses For the Noongar people's use of Eucalypts, see page 24.

Active Constituents For Eucalypts' active constituents, see page 24.

Family Myrtaceae Juss.

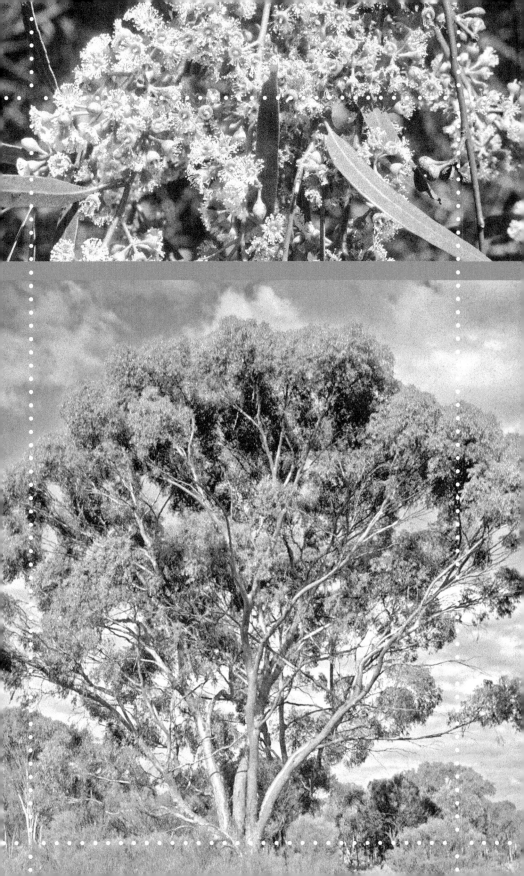

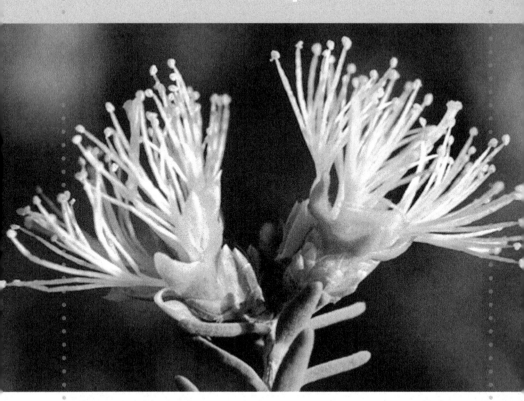

Family **Myrtaceae Juss.**

Botanical Name *Melaleuca cuticularis* Labill.

Common Name Saltwater Paperbark.

Noongar Names Bibool (WNRM, 2009), Bewel, Koll and Mudurda (Bindon & Chadwick, 2011).

Description Saltwater Paperbark grows as a shrub or tree to a height of 7 m. Archer (2016) relates that the main feature of the tree is its 'thick white flaky bark and the rugged gnarled and twisted tree growth'. The white, brush-like flowers appear from September to December (late Djilba to early Birak) (FloraBase, 2016).

Habitat Saltwater Paperbark grows in a variety of soils, including alluvium, sand and clay (FloraBase, 2016). It grows around both salt and fresh water near watercourses, lakes and swamps (Archer, 2016).

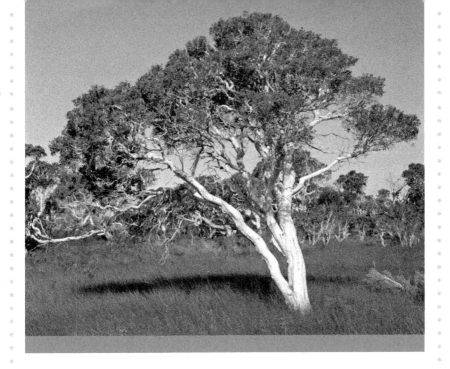

Distribution Saltwater Paperbark is native to Western Australia and is found mostly in coastal regions from Perth to Israelite Bay. It has also been sighted in the Avon Wheatbelt, on the Esperance Plains and in the Western Mallee (FloraBase, 2016).

Parts Used The leaves, timber and bark.

Medicinal Uses The leaves contain pleasant-smelling oils, similar to Eucalyptus oil, which Aboriginal people used in the treatment of colds. The bark of all paperbark species was used as bandages (Isaacs, 2009).

Other Uses Before colonisation, the bark was pulled off in large sheets to create clean surfaces for food, food and water containers and temporary shelters. The plant produces a hard, heavy, durable and termite-resistant timber that was probably used to make weapons and tools (Archer, 2016).

Active Constituents For Melaleucas' active constituents, see page 83.

Sandalwood

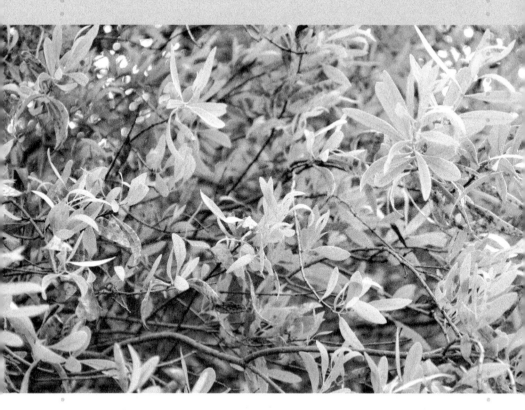

Family Santalaceae R.Br.

Botanical Name *Santalum spicatum* (R.Br.) A.DC.

Common Name Sandalwood.

Noongar Names Willarak, Uilarac, Waang, Wolgol and Wollgat (Abbott, 1983).

Description Sandalwood grows as a small tree up to 5 m in height. It is a parasitic plant which feeds off the roots of trees nearby, usually Acacias such as Jam Wattle. The grey-green leaves are oval shaped to lance shaped and are tapered at both ends. The flowers have four red petals and a green centre, and they occur from February to June (Bunuru to early Makuru). The orange fruits are spherical and about 30 mm in diameter. They have edible kernels with hard shells. The fruits are present from August to December (Djilba to early Birak) (Australian Plants Online, 2003; Florabank, 2016; FloraBase, 2016).

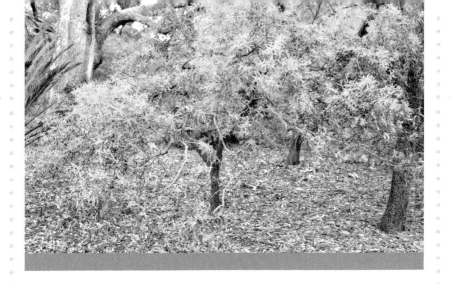

Habitat Sandalwood grows in a variety of soils and habitats including sandy, alkaline and limey-type soils on sandplains and among rocks (Florabank, 2016).

Distribution Sandalwood is found in the drier parts of the south-west of Western Australia southwards from Shark Bay and eastwards beyond Newman, Wiluna, Kalgoorlie and Norseman. It is also found in South Australia, from the border with Western Australia to the Flinders Ranges (Florabank, 2016). It used to grow around the Perth region but has been harvested to extinction in that area (Cunningham, 1998).

Parts Used The bark, nuts and leaves.

Medicinal Uses Decoctions of the inner bark were drunk as cough mixtures and to treat bronchitis. The oil from the nuts was used as a rubbing medicine to relieve colds and stiffness and on skin rashes (Lassak & McCarthy, 2001). The crushed leaves were applied as poultices to burns, scalds and sores (Cunningham, 1998).

Other Uses Smoke from the leaves was used ceremonially because of its powerful aroma (Cunningham, 1998).

Active Constituents Lassak and McCarthy (2001) report that the volatile wood oil is rich in santalol, which shows antibacterial activity. The active constituent in the leaves is not known.

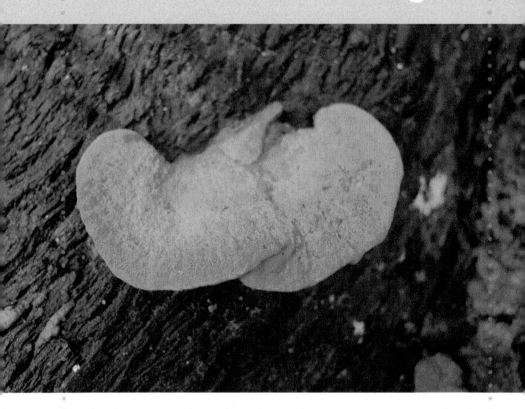

Family Coriolaceae.

Botanical Name *Pycnoporus coccineus* (Fr.) Bondartsev & Singer.

Common Names Scarlet Bracket Fungus and Orange Bracket Fungus.

Noongar Name Botting.

Description Scarlet Bracket Fungus is a bright orange, shelf-type fungus found on dead, decaying wood and occasionally on live trees. Its body may extend up to 60 mm beyond the wood and may grow up to 10 mm or so thick near the wood and thinner at the edges (ANBG, 2013; BRAIN, 2016).

Habitat Scarlet Bracket Fungus grows in a range of soils, habitats and conditions from the more moist, higher rainfall areas to much drier regions (BRAIN, 2016).

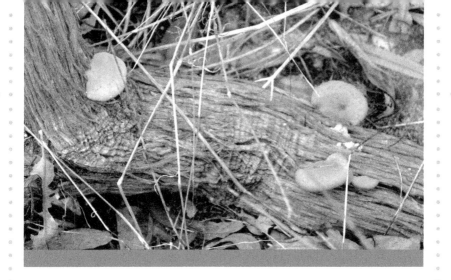

Distribution Scarlet Bracket Fungus is very widespread throughout southern Australia and into southern Queensland. In the south-west, it is found in coastal areas from Shark Bay to Israelite Bay (Atlas of Living Australia, 2016).

Parts Used The body of the fungus.

Medicinal Uses Aboriginal people used to rub pieces of Scarlet Bracket Fungus on the lips and in the mouths of babies and children to cure oral thrush and sore lips, and to relieve the symptoms of teething (ANBG, 2013).

Active Constituents The ANBG (2013) relates that the plant has been discovered to contain 'two antibiotic compounds'. Unfortunately, it does not name the compounds.

Caution
Bougher (2009) warns that a licence is needed to collect fungi on public land in Western Australia as fungi are a protected species.

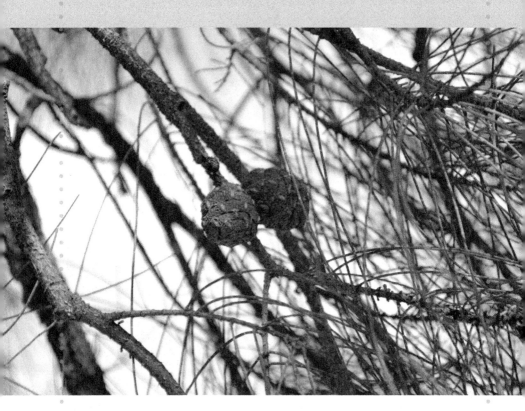

Family Casuarinaceae R.Br.

Botanical Name *Allocasuarina fraseriana* (Miq.) L.A.S.Johnson.

Common Names Sheoak, Western Sheoak and Common Sheoak.

Noongar Names Condil (Abbott, 1983), Kulli, Gulli (Bourne, 2016) and Kwell.

Description Sheoak is a tree that grows to a height of about 15 m, although it can be more stunted near the coast. It has slender, green cladodes (branchlets, or needles). Small, red, spiky male and female flowers appear on separate trees from May to October (late Djeran to early Kambarang). Small, egg-shaped cones appear after the flowers (Flora of Australia Online, 2016; FloraBase, 2016).

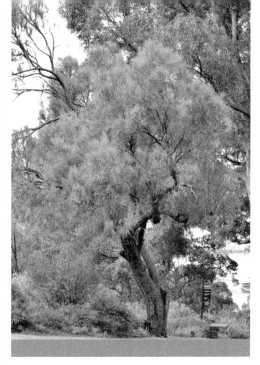

Habitat Sheoak prefers lateritic and sandy soils in forests and woodland areas (Flora of Australia Online, 2016).

Distribution Sheoak is native to the south-west of Western Australia and occurs in coastal and near-coastal areas in the south-west corner of the state, from Jurien Bay to Bremer Bay (Flora of Australia Online, 2016).

Parts Used The needle-like leaves.

Uses The Sheoak was vital to Noongar people's spirituality and social and emotional wellbeing. They sat under the tree and listened to the sounds of the breeze blowing through the foliage; they believed these were the whispers of the spirits of the old people talking to them. Babies were placed under the Sheoak to help induce sleep, as the sounds were believed to be the spirits of the old ones gently whispering to them to put them to sleep. Noongar people believed that when the Sheoak needles fell on their faces, they were tears of healing from the ancestors.

Noongar women often gave birth under the Sheoak because of the softness of the needles, which were also used for bedding in shelters, covered with kangaroo skins. This combination made very comfortable beds. The young cones were eaten (ANBG, 2016a).

Botanical Name *Cymbopogon obtectus* S.T.Blake.

Common Name Silky Heads.

Noongar Name Djiraly.

Description Silky Heads is a fragrant plant that grows to around 1 m in height. Its narrow leaves can be flat or folded. Its green-purple flowers have long, fluffy hairs. They appear in summer (Birak to early Bunuru) (RBGDT, 2016).

Habitat Silky Heads grows in a variety of soils, including sand, loam and granite, in arid and semi-arid areas (FloraBase, 2016).

Distribution Silky Heads grows across mainland Australia (Atlas of Living Australia, 2016). It occurs in most parts of Western Australia and has been sighted as far north as Halls Creek and beyond Kalgoorlie near the border with South Australia (FloraBase, 2016).

Parts Used The leaves and roots.

Medicinal Uses Decoctions of the crushed leaves were drunk to relieve coughs and colds; they were also used as liniment to ease sore muscles and headaches and as antiseptic on sores. Colds were treated with the crushed leaves held under the nose or placed in the nostrils. Decoctions of the roots were poured into the ear to relieve earaches (RBGDT, 2016).

Family Poaceae Barnhart & Barnh.

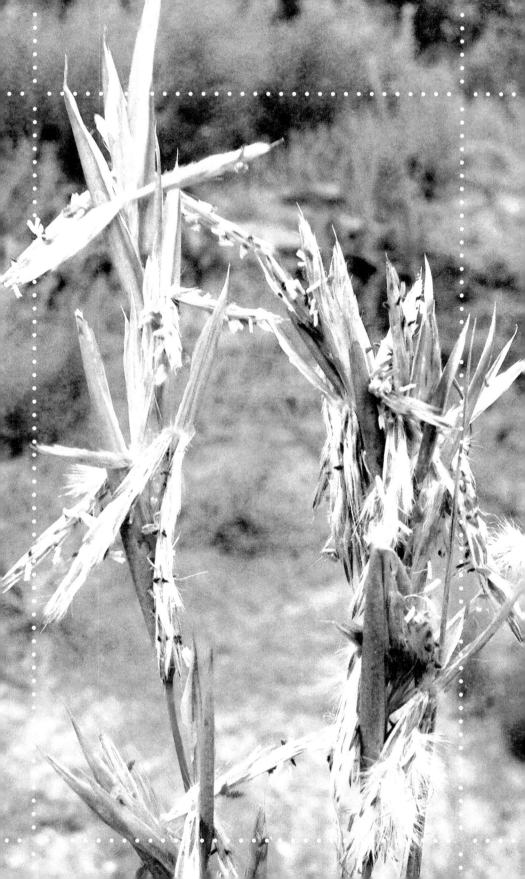

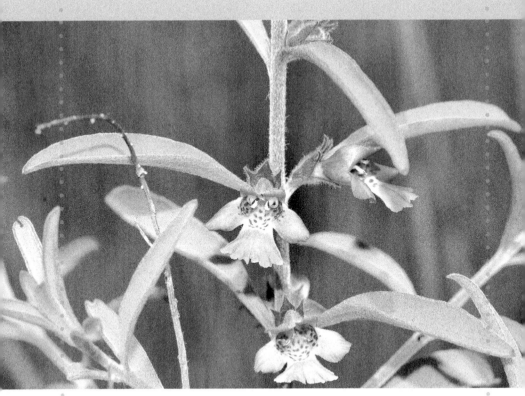

Family Lamiaceae Martinov.

Botanical Name *Hemigenia incana* (Lindl.) Benth.

Common Name Silky Hemigenia.

Noongar Names Not known for this plant.

Description Silky Hemigenia is a shrub that grows to around 1.4 m high. It has dark green leaves that are oval shaped and hairy. The blue to blue-purple, orchid-like flowers appear from August to November (Djilba to Kambarang) (ANBG, 2016b; FloraBase, 2016).

Habitat Silky Hemigenia grows in a range of habitats in loamy and gravelly laterite (FloraBase, 2016).

Distribution Silky Hemigenia is native to the south-west of Western Australia and is found in the moister regions from just north of Perth to Bremer Bay. It has been seen as far inland as Hyden (FloraBase, 2016).

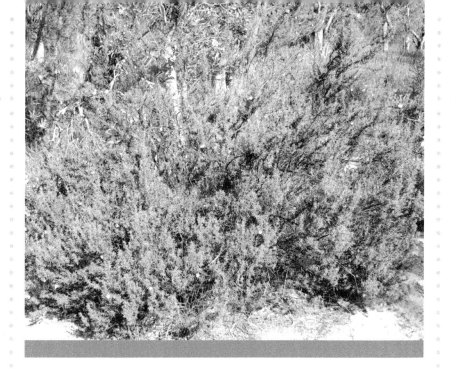

Parts Used The leaves and stems.

Medicinal Uses The leaves and stems were crushed and the vapours inhaled to treat headaches, colds and sinusitis. The leaves were mashed and applied to the body to soothe aches and pains.

Botanical Name *Eremophila scoparia* (R.Br.) F.Muell.

Common Names Silver Emu Bush, Scotia Bush and Broom Bush.

Noongar Name Barang.

Description Silver Emu Bush is a Broom bush that grows up to 3 m in height. It has narrow leaves and the stems are covered in grey scales that give the plant a silvery appearance (Archer, 2016). It can have blue, purple, pink or white tube-shaped flowers, which can appear at any time of the year but mainly from August to November (Djilba to Kambarang) (FloraBase, 2016). After flowering has finished, cone-shaped, dry, woody, scaly fruits appear (NSWFO, 2016).

Habitat Silver Emu Bush is found in various types of soils and habitats (FloraBase, 2016).

Distribution Silver Emu Bush is native to the southern areas of Australia. In Western Australia, it is found only on the outskirts of Noongar country from the Avon Wheatbelt to the South Australian border (FloraBase 2016). It grows quite prolifically around and to the north of Esperance (Archer, 2016).

Parts Used The leaves.

Medicinal Uses Decoctions of the leaves were used externally as washes for sores and were taken internally to treat colds, headaches, diarrhoea and chest pains.

Family Scrophulariaceae Juss.

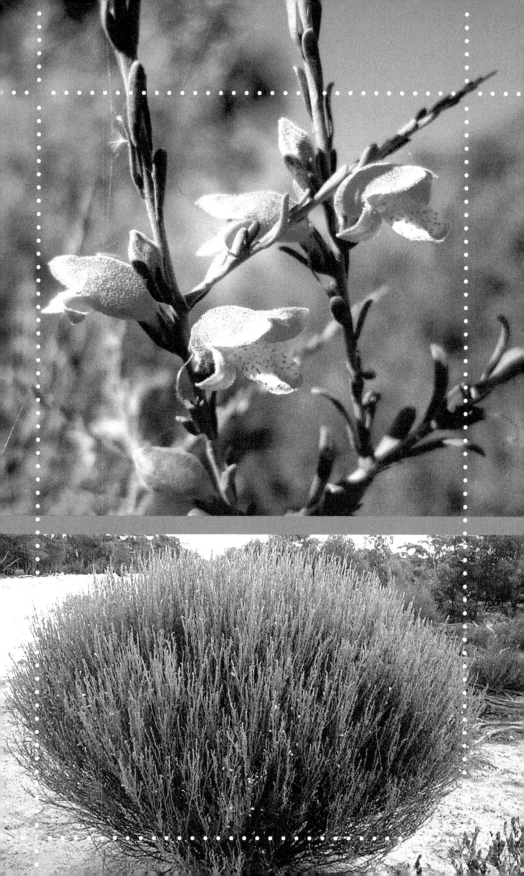

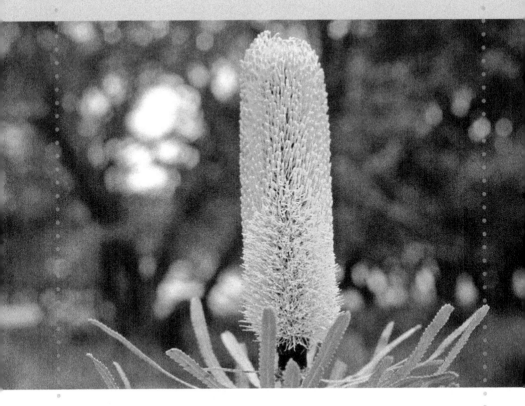

Botanical Name *Banksia attenuata* R.Br.

Common Names Slender Banksia, Candlestick Banksia and Coastal Banksia.

Noongar Names Piara, Biara, Bealwra, Peera, Piras (City of Joondalup, 2011) and Binda (Abbott, 1983).

Description Slender Banksia grows as a shrub or tree to around 10 m in height. It has long, narrow, serrated leaves around 250 mm in length and bright yellow, cylindrical flowers that look like large candlesticks. The flowers appear in spring and summer (late Djilba to early Bunuru). The tree has the ability to regenerate after a bushfire, thanks to its lignotuberous root system (Oz Native Plants, 2016).

Habitat Slender Banksia grows in sand in a variety of habitats (FloraBase, 2016).

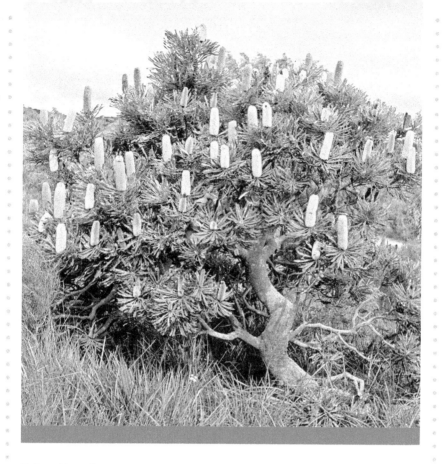

Distribution Slender Banksia is native to the south-west of Western Australia and is found across much of the south-west, from Kalbarri to Esperance and as far inland as the Avon Wheatbelt and the Western Mallee (FloraBase, 2016).

Uses For the Noongar people's use of Banksias, see page 16.

Small Leaf Clematis

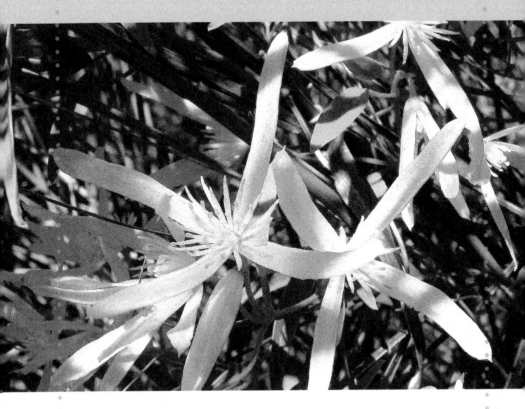

Family Ranunculaceae Juss.

Botanical Names *Clematis linearifolia* Steud., formerly *Clematis microphylla*.

Common Names Small Leaf Clematis, Small Clematis and Old Man's Beard (Lassak & McCarthy, 2001).

Noongar Name Taaruk.

Description Small Leaf Clematis is a climbing plant with wiry stems, which grow to around 5 m long. The plant is usually found draped over a small host shrub. It has long, narrow, oblong or lance-shaped leaves, which can grow up to 75 mm in length. The creamy-white, star-shaped flowers have four petals and spiky, long stamens. They appear from July to October (late Makuru to early Kambarang) (Archer, 2016; Flora of Australia Online, 2016).

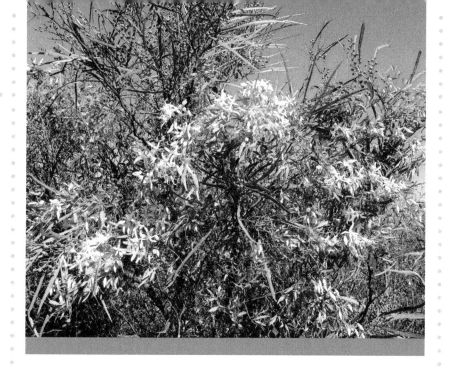

Habitat Small Leaf Clematis prefers sandy soils on sand dunes, in hollows and around lakes (Archer, 2016).

Distribution Small Leaf Clematis is found only on coastal sandplains in Western Australia, from Shark Bay to Augusta and around Esperance (FloraBase, 2016).

Parts Used The leaves.

Medicinal Uses Poultices of the crushed leaves were applied to irritated skin.

Caution
Lassak and McCarthy (2001) warn that poultices made from *Clematis* species should not be left on the skin for more than 3 minutes, as it could have the opposite effect from that intended and cause more irritation and even blistering.

Botanical Name *Hydrocotyle callicarpa* Bunge.

Common Names Small Pennywort and Tiny Pennywort.

Noongar Names Not known for this plant.

Description Small Pennywort is diminutive annual herb that grows only to around 80 mm high. The little, light green, hairy leaves have three or five lobes. The tiny white, yellow or purple flowers appear from August to November (Djilba to Kambarang). They are clustered on stalks 2–10 mm long (FloraBase, 2016; NSWFO, 2016).

Habitat Small Pennywort prefers sandy and lateritic soils in a variety of habitats including moist, winter-wet areas, rocky outcrops and limestone crests (FloraBase, 2016).

Distribution Small Pennywort is native to the south-west of Western Australia and is found all over that area. It also grows in the southern reaches of South Australia and New South Wales and throughout Victoria and Tasmania (Atlas of Living Australia, 2016).

Parts Used The leaves.

Medicinal Uses The leaves were burnt and the smoke inhaled to treat rheumatic pain. Fresh leaves were crushed and the vapours inhaled to relieve headaches and colds; they were also chewed to relieve toothache.

Family Araliaceae Juss.

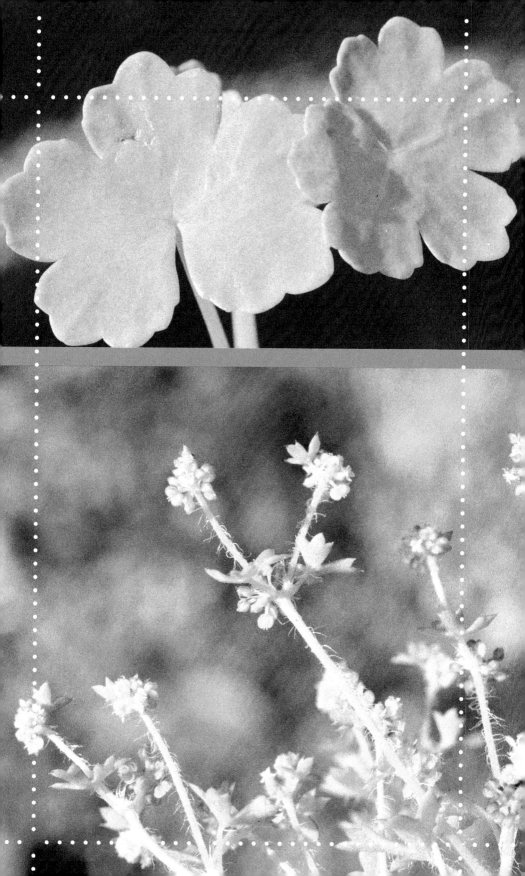

Snottygobble

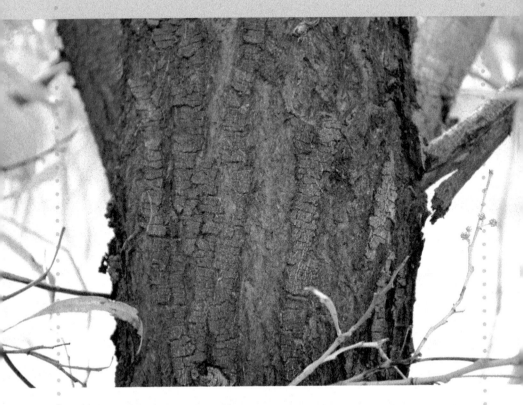

Family Proteaceae Juss.

Botanical Name *Persoonia longifolia* R.Br.

Common Name Snottygobble.

Noongar Name Kadgeegurr.

Description Snottygobble grows as an erect shrub or tree to about 5 m in height. Its rough, flaky bark is a dark red colour, with deep, vertical grooves on the trunk. The dark green leaves are long, narrow and slightly elliptical, and they grow to around 220 mm in length. The yellow-orange flowers appear from November to February (late Kambarang to early Bunuru). The spherical fruits appear in summer and autumn (Birak to Djeran) and are green initially but turn yellow as they ripen (Perth Seed, 2010).

Habitat Snottygobble prefers sand, sandy loam and laterite in coastal and near coastal habitats (FloraBase, 2016).

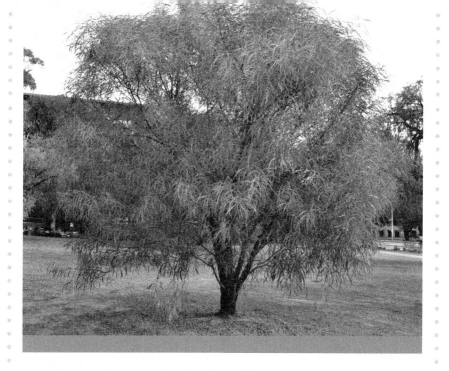

Distribution Snottygobble is native to the south-west of Western Australia. It grows in coastal and near-coastal areas from Perth to Albany (FloraBase, 2016).

Parts Used The bark and leaves.

Medicinal Uses Decoctions of the bark were applied externally to relieve skin disorders and as eyewashes. Infusions of the leaves were taken internally to relieve colds and sore throats.

Other Uses The fruits were eaten as food. The flesh resembles snot, or mucous – hence the name. It is thought that Noongars sucked the seeds of the Snottygobble on long treks to keep the mouth moist and to avert thirst (Perth Seed, 2010).

Spearwood Mallee

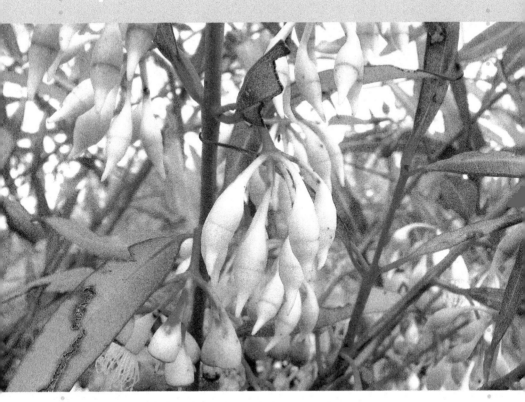

Botanical Name *Eucalyptus doratoxylon* F.Muell.

Common Names Spearwood Mallee and Bell Gum.

Noongar Name Geitch-gmunt (Abbott, 1983).

Description Spearwood Mallee is a Eucalypt that grows to around 6 m in height. Its multiple trunks are powdery white when young, but as the plant matures they develop rough, flaky bark at their bases, leaving only the upper branches smooth and white. The leaves are medium to dark green, long, narrow and lance shaped. The white flowers can appear at almost any time of the year, with the main period being from August to January (Djilba to Birak). The plant is able to recover after a bushfire due to its lignotuberous root system (Archer, 2016; FloraBase, 2016).

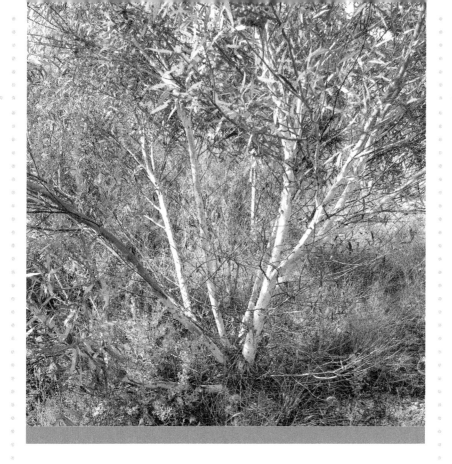

Habitat Spearwood Mallee prefers sandy soils on granite ridges and hillsides (Florabase, 2016).

Distribution Spearwood Mallee is native to the southern reaches of the south-west of Western Australia. It is found only in coastal and near-coastal areas near Albany and Esperance (Archer, 2016; FloraBase, 2016).

Parts Used The leaves, gum and wood.

Medicinal Uses For Eucalypts' medicinal uses, see page 24.

Other Uses Noongars of the south coast used the branches for spear making. Bends in the shaft of the spear would be straightened out over a fire and the tips sharpened with a chert flake (a silica rich rock) (Archer, 2016).

Active Constituents For Eucalypts' active constituents, see page 24.

Starflower

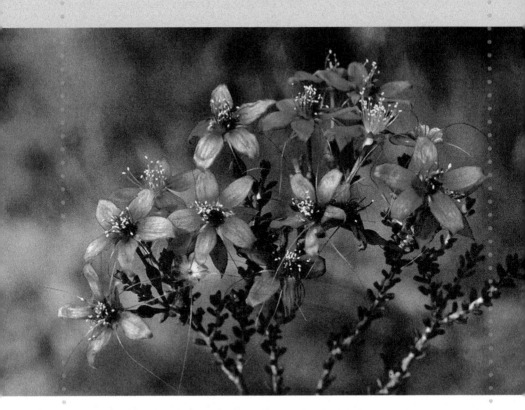

Botanical Name *Calytrix strigosa* A.Cunn.

Common Name Starflower.

Noongar Name Koorin.

Description Starflower is a small shrub that grows only to around 1.6 m in height, with a spread of about 1 m. The tiny leaves are about 5 mm long. The large, star-shaped flowers have five petals and can be pink, purple or yellow in colour. They appear from late winter to early summer (late Djilba to early Birak) (ANPSA, 2016; FloraBase, 2016).

Habitat Starflower prefers sand and laterite and is found mostly on sandplains (FloraBase, 2016).

Distribution Starflower is native to the south-west of Western Australia. It grows from Carnarvon across the

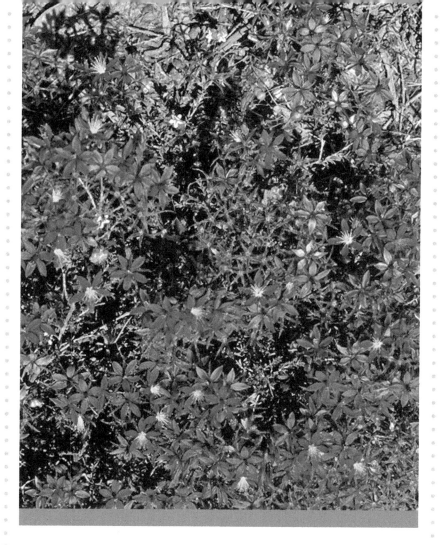

Geraldton Sandplains and the Avon Wheatbelt and along the coastal plain to just south of Perth (FloraBase, 2016).

Parts Used The bark, leaves and twigs.

Medicinal Uses Infusions of the bark, leaves and twigs were applied externally to treat skin problems. The crushed bark mixed with oil or fat was rubbed around the neck and nose to relieve sinusitis. The mashed leaves were used externally as liniment to ease rheumatic conditions, muscle aches, bruises, sprains and small wounds.

Botanical Name *Goodenia varia* R.Br.

Common Names Sticky Goodenia and Kalgoorlie Honey Dew.

Noongar Names Not known for this plant.

Description Sticky Goodenia is a small, prostrate shrub that grows to around 0.6 m in height. It has thick leaves, which are slightly toothed and have a sticky texture – hence the name. The tiny, almost elliptical, yellow flowers have five petals and appear from October to November (Kambarang) (Customary Medicinal Knowledgebase, 2011; Lassak & McCarthy, 2001).

Habitat Sticky Goodenia prefers sand and clay. It is found in a variety of habitats, including coastal limestone cliffs and sand dunes (FloraBase, 2016).

Distribution Sticky Goodenia is native to Western Australia. In Noongar country, it is found along the south coast from Albany to beyond Esperance. It is also found in southern South Australia and Victoria (Atlas of Living Australia, 2016).

Part Used The leaves.

Medicinal Uses Decoctions of the leaves were taken internally as a sedative. Lassak and McCarthy (2001) believe that the sedatives were safe for children, as Aboriginal mothers were thought to use a small amount to 'pacify children on long and arduous journeys'.

Family Goodeniaceae R.Br.

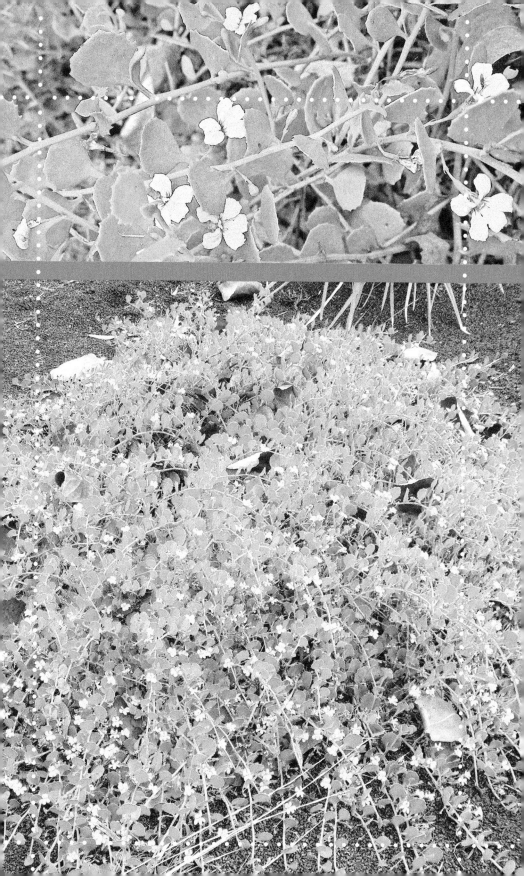

Sticky Hopbush

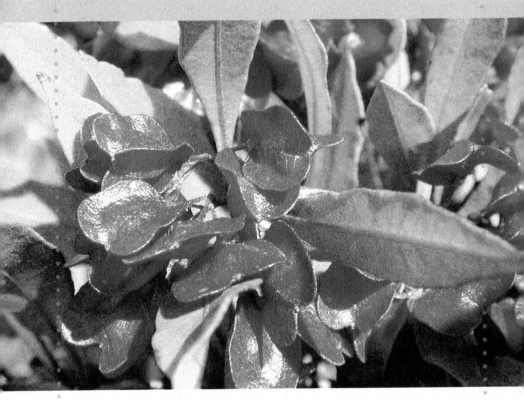

Family Sapindaceae Juss.

Botanical Names *Dodonaea viscosa* Jacq., synonyms *Dodonaea angustifolia*, *Dodonaea attenuate* A.Cunn.

Common Names Sticky Hopbush, Desert Hopbush, Broad Leaf Hopbush, Candlewood, Narrow Leaf Hopbush, Native Hopbush, Soapwood, Switch Sorrel, Wedge Leaf Hopbush, Native Hop, Giant Hopbush and Hopbush.

Noongar Name Waning (Abbott, 1983).

Other Aboriginal Names Watchupga, Kirni and Tecan (Lassak & McCarthy, 2001).

Description Sticky Hopbush is an evergreen shrub or small tree that grows to about 5 m in height. The sticky leaves vary in shape from elliptical to oblong and are reddish or purplish in colour (Lassak & McCarthy, 2001). In Western Australia its

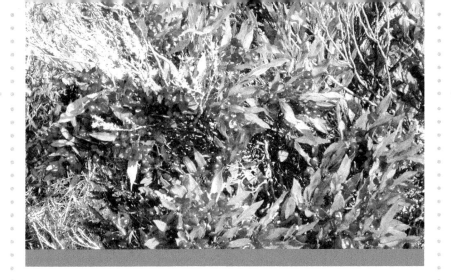

greenish-yellow flowers appear from June to August (Makuru to early Djilba) (FloraBase, 2016).

Habitat Sticky Hopbush prefers sand, loam and clay. It grows in arid and semi-arid areas in a variety of habitats (FloraBase, 2016).

Distribution Sticky Hopbush is found throughout mainland Australia as well as in Africa and throughout Europe, the Pacific Islands and the Americas (Cribb & Cribb, 1983). It grows across the south-west of Western Australia (FloraBase, 2016).

Parts Used The leaves and roots.

Medicinal Uses The leaves were chewed to soothe toothache, though the juice was not swallowed (Lassak & McCarthy, 2001). The crushed leaves and the juice were used externally in the treatment of stonefish and stingray wounds. The juice of the crushed leaves is also reported to have antifungal and anti-inflammatory properties (Venkatesh et al., 2008). Infusions of the leaves were rubbed all over the body to reduce fevers.

Other Uses The leafy branches produce clean smoke, which was used to smoke babies, in smoking ceremonies to keep out bad spirits, and as insect repellent.

Straggly Mallee

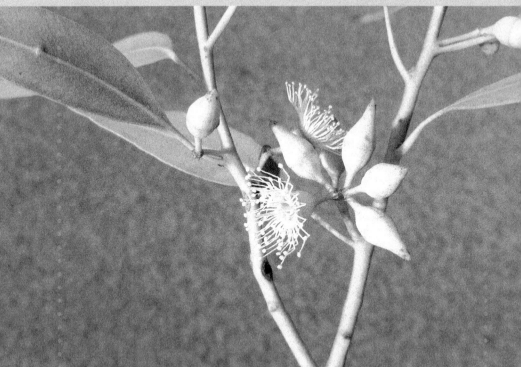

Family Myrtaceae Juss.

Botanical Name *Eucalyptus petrensis* Brooker & Hopper.

Common Names Straggly Mallee and Limestone Mallee.

Noongar Name Koojat (City of Joondalup, 2011).

Description Straggly Mallee is a Eucalypt that grows to 4 m high. It has smooth bark and ovate leaves with pointy ends. The spiky, white flowers appear from June to October (Makuru to early Kambarang) (FloraBase, 2016).

Habitat Straggly Mallee prefers sand over coastal limestone (FloraBase, 2016).

Distribution Straggly Mallee is native to and is found exclusively on the Geraldton Sandplains, the Central West Coast plain and the Swan Coastal Plain in the south-west of Western Australia (FloraBase, 2016).

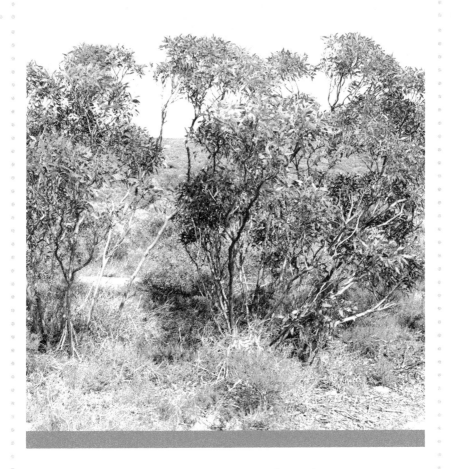

Uses For the Noongar people's use of Eucalypts, see page 24.

Active Constituents For Eucalypts' active constituents, see page 24.

Swamp Banksia

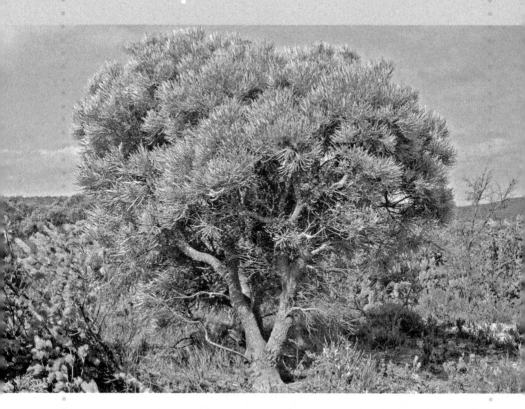

Botanical Name *Banksia littoralis* R.Br.

Common Names Swamp Banksia, Swamp Oak and Western Swamp Banksia.

Noongar Names Pungura (Bennett, 1991), Boora, Boorarup and Mimidi.

Description Swamp Banksia grows as a large shrub or tree up to 20 m in height. The bark is grey and quite rough. The long, lance-shaped leaves are dark green with toothed edges and grow to around 200 mm in length. The bright orange-yellow flowers are cylindrical spikes around 200 mm long. They appear from March to August (late Bunuru to early Djilba) (FloraBase, 2016; Oz Native Plants, 2016).

Habitat Swamp Banksia is found in peaty sand in low-lying, damp areas near rivers, swamps and lakes (FloraBase, 2016).

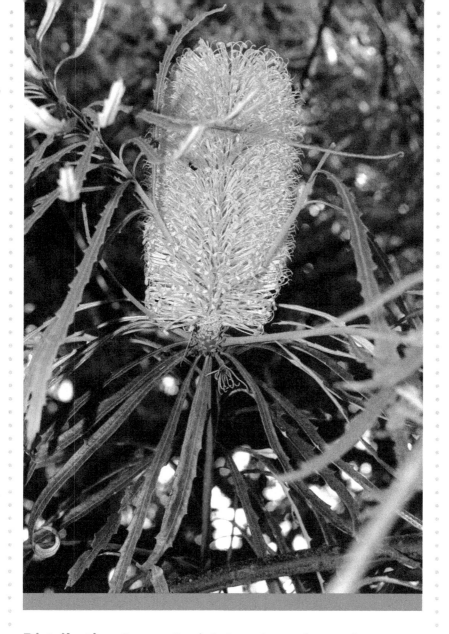

Distribution Swamp Banksia is native to the south-west of Western Australia and is found throughout this area from Lancelin to Bremer Bay and as far inland as the Avon Wheatbelt. It is also found on the Esperance Plains and the Geraldton Sandplains (FloraBase, 2016).

Uses For the Noongar people's use of Banksias, see page 16.

Botanical Name *Eucalyptus patens* Benth.

Common Names Swan River Blackbutt, Western Australian Blackbutt and Yarri.

Noongar Name Dwutta (Abbott, 1983).

Description Swan River Blackbutt is usually a tall tree growing up to 45 m in height but can be shorter in swampy areas. The almost-black, longitudinally furrowed bark is where its name originates. The glossy, medium green leaves are long and lance shaped. The white or cream flowers appear from July to August (late Makuru to early Djilba) or from November to December (late Kambarang to early Birak) (FloraBase, 2016).

Habitat Swan River Blackbutt grows in a variety of soils, including sand, gravel, clay and loam. It is mostly found in moist depressions and along watercourses (FloraBase, 2016).

Distribution Swan River Blackbutt grows in coastal and near-coastal areas from just north of Perth to Albany (FloraBase, 2016).

Uses For the Noongar people's use of Eucalypts, see page 24.

Active Constituents For Eucalypts' active constituents, see page 24.

Family **Myrtaceae Juss.**

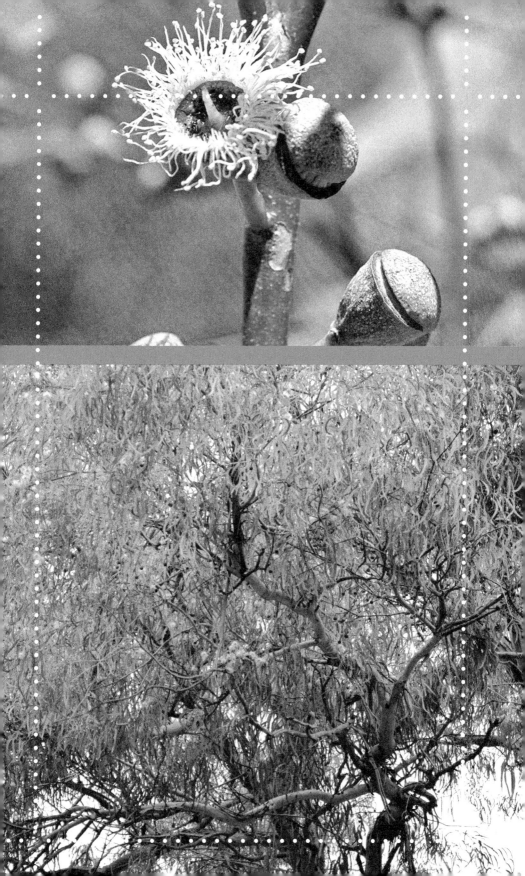

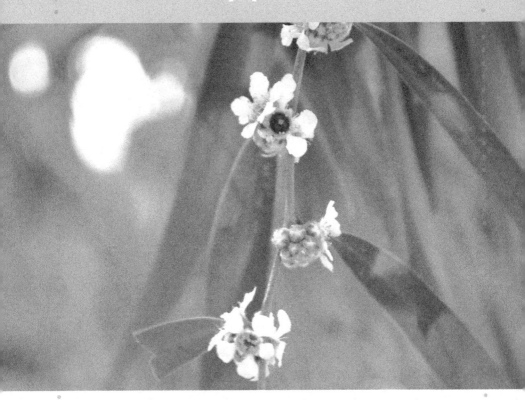

Botanical Name *Agonis flexuosa* (Willd.) Sweet.

Common Names Sweet Peppermint and Willow Myrtle.

Noongar Names Wanil, Wanill, Wannow, Wonong (Abbott, 1983), Wannung and Warndilyy (Bindon & Chadwick, 2011).

Description Sweet Peppermint is a tree with a graceful, weeping habit and grows to around 15 m in height or more in good conditions. It has fibrous, longitudinally furrowed, rough bark and long, narrow, lance-shaped leaves. Its white flowers, which have five petals, appear in spring and summer (late Djilba to early Bunuru) and form bunched up clusters along the thin branches (ANPSA, 2016).

Habitat Sweet Peppermint prefers sand and laterite in coastal and near-coastal areas (FloraBase, 2016).

Family Myrtaceae Juss.

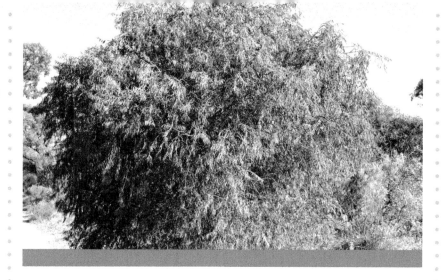

Distribution Sweet Peppermint is native to the south-west of Western Australia. It is found in coastal and near-coastal situations from Perth to beyond Bremer Bay (FloraBase, 2016). It is the most prolific tree of the Swan Coastal Plain and can be seen in large numbers around the Perth area, both in natural bushland and in domestic settings, on verges and in parks.

Parts Used The leaves, twigs and gum.

Medicinal Uses Mothers crushed the leaves between their palms and then placed their hot, peppermint-scented hands on the chests of babies to ease chest and nasal congestion. Decoctions of the leaves were used as antiseptic washes on minor wounds and as mouthwashes. The smoke from the twigs and leaves was used to treat respiratory problems, and the ash from burnt twigs and leaves was mixed with fat and used as salves or poultices to treat wounds and sores.

Other Uses The leaves and gum were used ceremonially, and the twigs and leaves were used in smoking ceremonies. Young plants were made into spear shafts and digging sticks (*wanna*) (Bourne, 2016).

Active Constituents Studies in India have isolated the presence of myrcene, α-thujene and limonene as the major constituents in the essential oil (Saj & Thoppil, 2011).

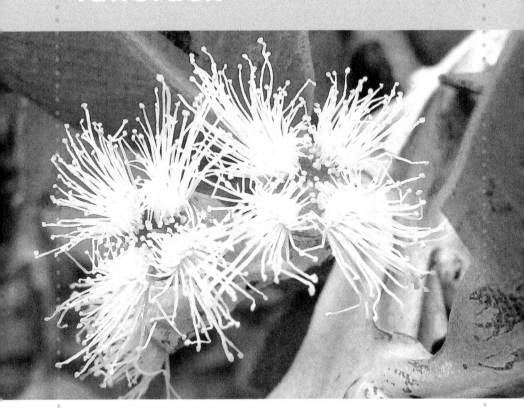

Botanical Names *Eucalyptus pleurocarpa* Schauer, formerly *Eucalyptus tetragona*.

Common Name Tallerack.

Noongar Name Tallerack (French, 2012).

Description Tallerack is a mallee Eucalypt that grows to around 4 m in height in coastal areas and up to 8 m in mallee (drier) regions. It usually has several bare trunks, and the foliage is normally restricted to the upper parts of the tree. According to Archer (2016), it 'is readily identified by the glaucous foliage, stems, buds and fruits that glow pale blue and white even from a distance'. The leaves are light green and quite oval shaped. The spiky, white flowers appear from November to February (late Kambarang to early Bunuru). The large, white, square fruits are present over several months (Archer, 2016).

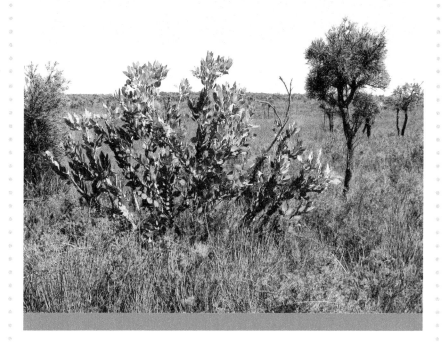

Habitat Tallerack grows in a variety of soils including sand, gravel and limestone. It is found on sandplains and in woodland areas including Jarrah forests (Archer, 2016; FloraBase, 2016).

Distribution Tallerack is native to the south coastal area of the south-west of Western Australia and is a very common species on the sandplain between Esperance and Albany (Archer, 2016).

Uses For the Noongar people's use of Eucalypts, see page 24.

Active Constituents For Eucalypts' active constituents, see page 24.

Botanical Name *Melaleuca teretifolia* Endl.

Common Names Teatree, Marsh Honey Myrtle and Banbar.

Noongar Name Banbar.

Description Teatree is a shrub or small tree that can reach 5 m in height. Its needle-like leaves grow to around 60 mm long and have sharp, pointy ends. The white, cream or pink flowers occur in globe-shaped clusters from October to December (Kambarang to early Birak) or from January to March (late Birak to Bunuru) (ANPSA, 2016; FloraBase, 2016).

Habitat Teatree prefers sand and clay in and around swampy and seasonally wet areas (FloraBase, 2016).

Distribution Teatree is native to and grows naturally only in the south-west of Western Australia. It is found in coastal and near-coastal areas around Geraldton and from Perth to Busselton (FloraBase, 2016).

Parts Used The leaves and bark.

Medicinal Uses The leaves were crushed and the vapour inhaled to treat headaches and colds. Infusions of the leaves were drunk to relieve colds, congestion and headaches and were applied externally to skin problems and wounds. The bark was soaked and applied to wounds as an anti-inflammatory.

Active Constituents For Melaleucas' active constituents, see page 83.

Family Myrtaceae Juss.

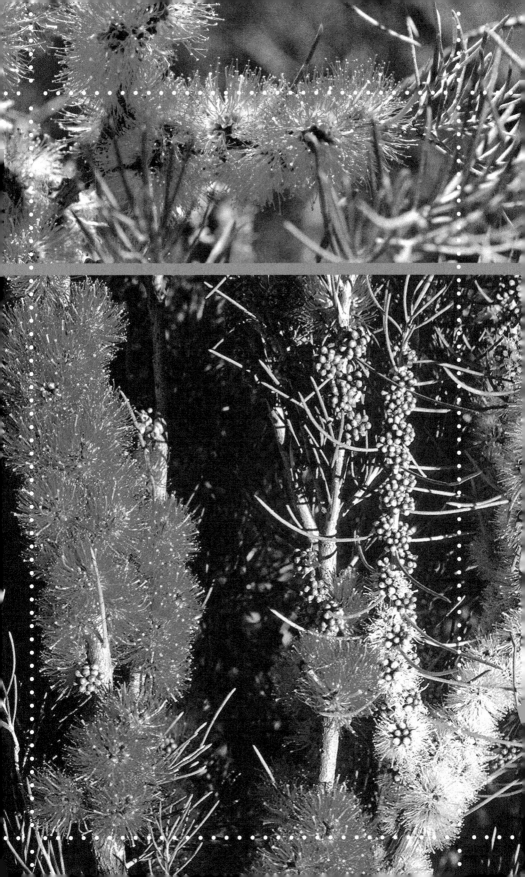

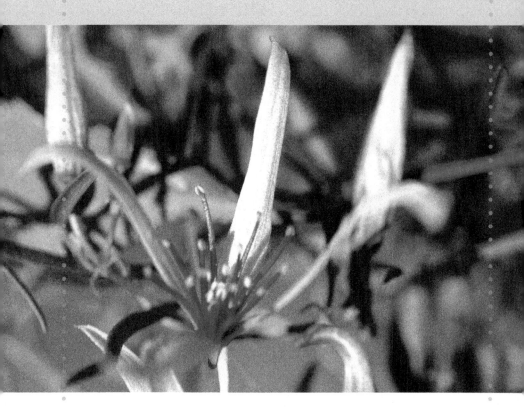

Botanical Name *Clematis delicata* W.T.Wang.

Common Names Toothache Bush and Delicate Clematis.

Noongar Names Not known for this plant.

Description Toothache Bush is a creeper or weak climber that grows to around 2 m in height. It typically has narrow, needle-like leaf blades. Its delicate flowers have five thin petals and are white with shades of pink or purple. The flowers appear from July to September (late Makuru to Djilba) (Atlas of Living Australia, 2016; FloraBase, 2016).

Habitat Toothache Bush prefers sand (FloraBase, 2016). It grows in dry, open forests, woodlands and mallee scrubs (Flora of Australia Online, 2016).

Distribution Toothache Bush is native solely to Western Australia and grows only in the south-west of the state. It has

Family **Ranunculaceae.**

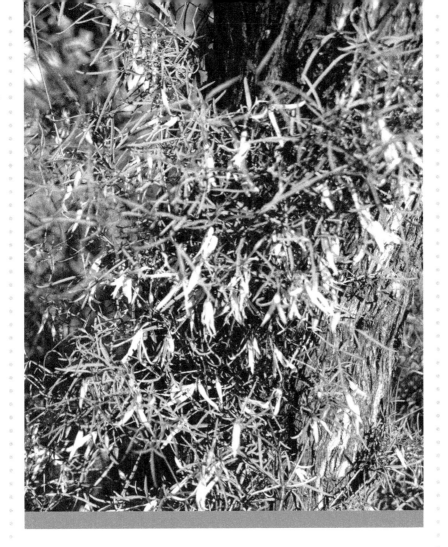

been sighted from Geraldton and inland through the Avon Wheatbelt and the Western Mallee to the Esperance Plains (FloraBase, 2016).

Parts Used The leaves.

Medicinal Uses When chewed, the leaves numb the mouth and gums and were used to relieve toothache.

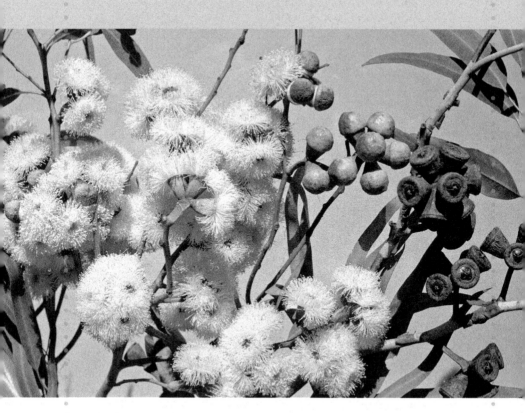

Botanical Name *Eucalyptus gomphocephala* DC.

Common Name Tuart.

Noongar Names Morrol, Duart, Mooarn, Moorun, Mouarn, Tuart and Tooart (Abbott, 1983; City of Joondalup, 2011).

Description Tuart is a tall, evergreen Eucalyptus tree that usually grows to 40 m in height; however, shorter, mallee forms have been seen in some areas north of Perth (Florabank, 2016). The bark is quite rough. White flowers appear from January to April (late Birak to early Djeran) (FloraBase, 2016).

Habitat Tuart thrives in sand over limestone on coastal sandplains (FloraBase, 2016).

Distribution Tuart is native to the south-west of Western Australia and occurs along a narrow limestone belt on the

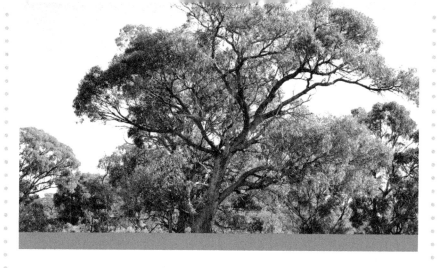

coastal plain north and south of Perth. Its natural range extends from Cape Naturalist to Cervantes (FloraBase, 2016).

Parts Used The leaves, gum and bark.

Medicinal Uses The gum was used as a mild anaesthetic, and large pieces were also used as fillings in dental cavities (City of Joondalup, 2011). For Eucalypts' other medicinal uses, see page 24.

Other Uses The bark was often used by Noongar people as roofing for shelters (City of Joondalup, 2011).

Active Constituents For Eucalypts' active constituents, see page 24.

Umbrella Bush

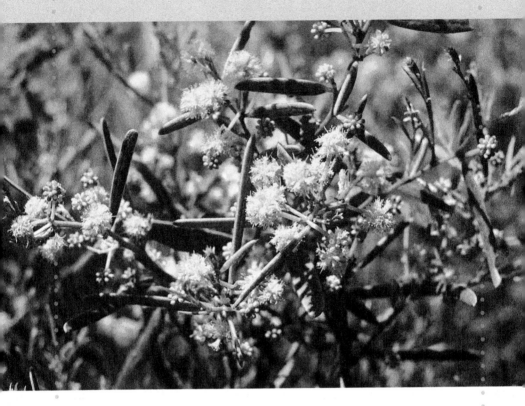

Family Fabaceae Lindl.

Botanical Names *Acacia ligulata* Benth., synonyms *Acacia bivenosa* subsp. *wayi*, *Acacia salicina* var. *wayi*.

Common Names Umbrella Bush, Small Cooba, Sandhill Wattle, Marpoo, Dune Wattle, and Wirra.

Noongar Names Not known for this plant.

Other Aboriginal Name Watarrka (Central Desert) (Bindon, 1996).

Description Umbrella Bush is a Wattle that grows as a shrub or small tree to around 4 m in height. It is sometimes dome shaped but often branches from the ground. The bark is usually grooved at the base but smooth further up. The narrow, oblong-shaped leaves, which are actually phyllodes, are light green to blue-green in colour and grow to around 100 mm long. The yellow to orange, globular flowers appear along the stems

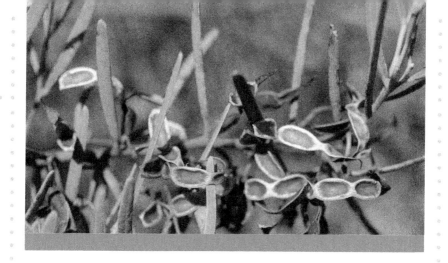

between the leaves from May to October (late Djeran to early Kambarang). The curved seed pods are light brown and grow to around 100 mm in length (Bindon, 1996; FloraBase, 2016).

Habitat Umbrella Bush prefers dry, alkaline soils and is found on coastal sand dunes (Lassak and McCarthy, 2001).

Distribution Umbrella Bush is native to Western Australia, South Australia and north-eastern Victoria. It is found in the drier parts of the south-west of Western Australia and along the southern coast from Albany to the South Australian border (Bindon, 1996). It also occurs in southern parts of the Northern Territory, in South Australia and in the drier regions of southern Queensland, New South Wales and Victoria (Florabank, 2016).

Parts Used The bark.

Medicinal Uses Infusions or decoctions of the bark were used as cough medicines and as washes for burns. Bindon (1996) relates that decoctions of the bark were also used as general treatment for dizziness, nerves and seizures and that the branches were used to smoke people suffering from general sickness and women following childbirth.

Other Uses The seeds were ground and eaten (Bindon, 1996). Grubs that inhabited the root system were eaten, raw or roasted. The shrub was also burnt and the ash mixed with the Native Tobacco, or Pituri (*Duboisia hopwoodii*), for chewing (Lassak & McCarthy, 2001).

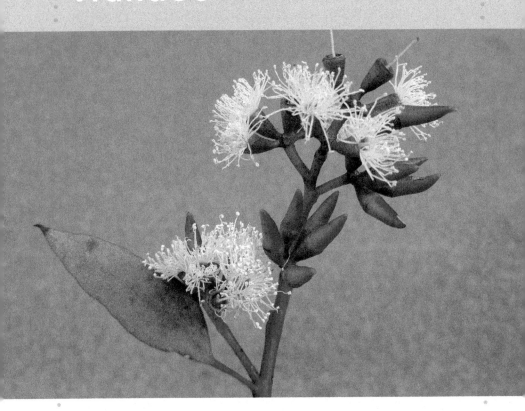

Botanical Name *Eucalyptus wandoo* Blakely.

Common Names Wandoo and White Gum.

Noongar Names Wornt, Dooto, Wando, Wandoo and Warrnt (Abbott, 1983).

Description Wandoo is a tall Eucalypt that grows to around 25 m in height. Its smooth bark is a mottled white colour. The lance-shaped leaves grow to around 120 mm in length, and white-cream, spiky flowers appear from December to May (Birak to Djeran) (FloraBase, 2016).

Habitat Wandoo grows in a variety of soils, sand, clay loam, gravel and laterite. It is found mostly on stony slopes and undulating ground (FloraBase, 2016).

Distribution Wandoo is native to the south-west of Western Australia. It is found throughout the south-west

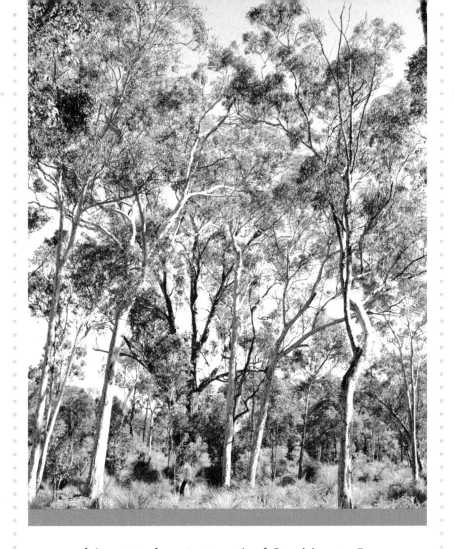

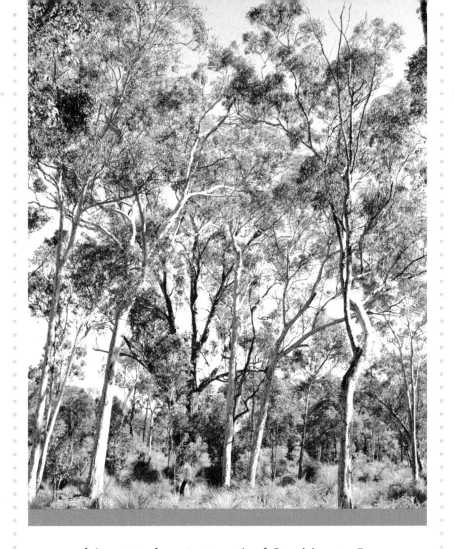

corner of the state, from just south of Geraldton to Bremer Bay and east to the Avon Wheatbelt and the Western Mallee (FloraBase, 2016).

Parts Used The leaves, gum, flowers and roots.

Medicinal Uses For Eucalypts' medicinal uses, see page 24.

Other Uses The sweet and juicy outer parts of the roots were scraped off and eaten. The flowers were soaked in water and made into a sweet drink (Coppin, 2008).

Active Constituents For Eucalypts' active constituents, see page 24.

Weeping Pittosporum

Botanical Name *Pittosporum angustifolium* Lodd.

Common Names Weeping Pittosporum, Butterbush, Native Willow, Poison Berry Tree, Cattle Bush and Native Apricot (Lassak & McCarthy, 2001).

Noongar Name Wongin.

Other Aboriginal Name Meemee (Cribb & Cribb, 1981).

Description Weeping Pittosporum grows as a weeping shrub or tree to around 8 m high. The leaves vary in shape from ovate to elliptic and can reach 85 mm in length. The white or cream, bell-shaped flowers appear from June to October (Makuru to early Kambarang). They are followed by smooth, yellow to orange fruits about 10–15 mm long (Cribb & Cribb, 1981; FloraBase, 2016).

Habitat Weeping Pittosporum prefers clay, sand and laterite near watercourses (FloraBase, 2016).

Distribution Weeping Pittosporum occurs from Geraldton to Perth and inland across the southern part of Western Australia. It also grows on Rottnest, Garden and Penguin islands (FloraBase, 2016; Rippey & Rowland, 1995).

Parts Used The seeds, fruits, leaves and wood.

Medicinal Uses Infusions of the seeds, fruit pulp, leaves or wood were taken internally for the relief of pain and cramps. Decoctions of the fruit pulp were drunk and applied externally to treat eczema and skin itches.

Other Uses A compress of warmed leaves was used to induce the flow of milk in new mothers (Peile, 1997).

Active Constituents Lassak and McCarthy (2001) report that 'the fruits and leaves contain a haemolytic saponin hydrolysing to the triterpenoid compounds pittosapogenin (R1-barrigenol) and phillyrigenin'.

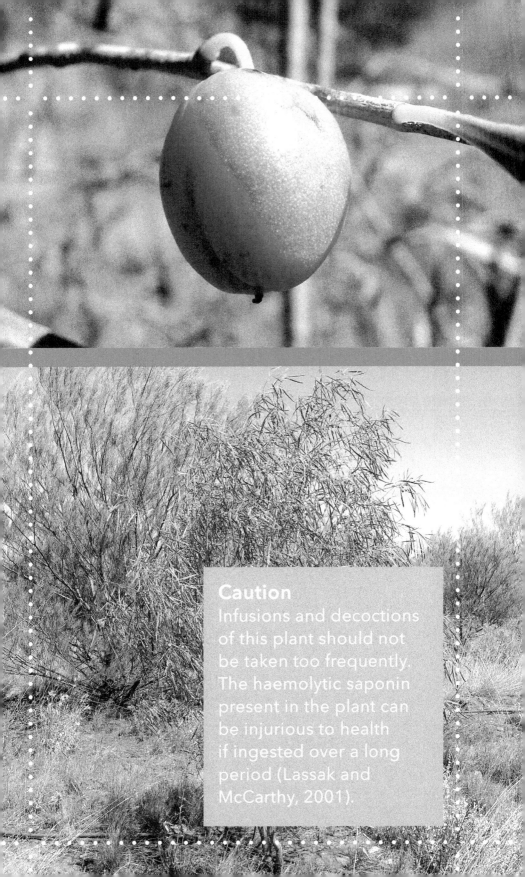

Caution
Infusions and decoctions
of this plant should not
be taken too frequently.
The haemolytic saponin
present in the plant can
be injurious to health
if ingested over a long
period (Lassak and
McCarthy, 2001).

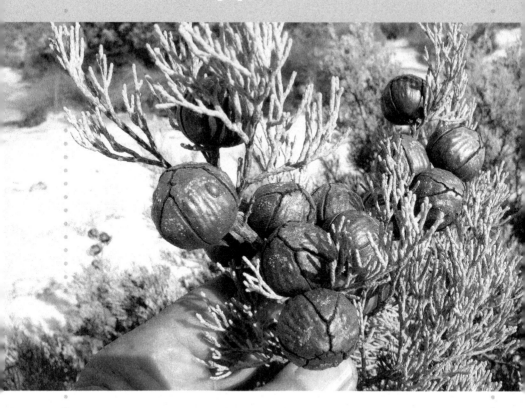

Family Cuppressaceae Gray.

Botanical Name *Callitris columellaris* F.Muell.

Common Name White Cypress Pine.

Noongar Names Not known for this plant.

Description White Cypress Pine is a small, evergreen, cone-shaped tree that usually grows to around 12 m but can be found up to 18 m in some parts of Australia. It has rough, vertically grooved bark and scale-like, blue-green leaves about 6 mm long, which twirl around the branchlets. The dark brown, spherical, woody cones are roughly 10–20 mm in diameter (FloraBase, 2016; Lassak & McCarthy, 2001).

Habitat White Cypress Pine grows in a variety of soils, including sandy and clay and loam, gravel and laterite. It is found growing in a variety of habitats including on sandplains, hillsides, in valleys, on clifftops and around salt lakes (FloraBase, 2016).

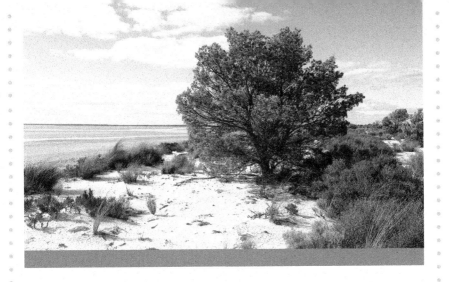

Distribution White Cypress Pine is native to Western Australia but is found throughout all of mainland Australia (Lassak & McCarthy, 2001). It grows in most parts of Western Australia, from the Northern Kimberley southwards. In the south-west of Western Australia, it occurs near the coast around Geraldton and in the drier inland areas from Geraldton to Esperance (FloraBase, 2016).

Parts Used The twigs, leaves and bark.

Medicinal Uses Infusions of the herb were used as chest rubs to treat colds and coughs and as washes for burns and insect bites. The leaves, bark and twigs were crushed and mixed with animal fat and rubbed on the chest to relieve congestion. They also made a good smoke medicine (Peile, 1997).

Active Constituents According to Lassak and McCarthy (2001), the resin contains several diterpenoid acids. Whether these are the active medicinal constituents is not known.

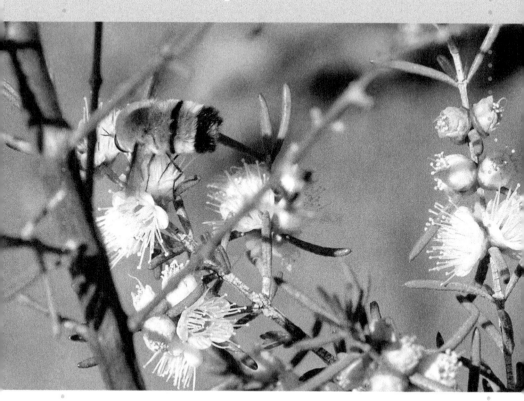

Botanical Name *Hypocalymma angustifolium*
(Endl.) Schauer.

Common Name White Myrtle.

Noongar Names Koodgeed and Kudjidi (Abbott, 1983).

Description White Myrtle is an erect shrub that grows
to about 1.5 m in height. It has very thin leaves, which are
about 25 mm long. The small, white or pink flowers appear
along the stems in small bunches of two or three from June
to October (Makuru to early Kambarang). Some flowers are
both white and pink (ANPSA, 2016; FloraBase, 2016).

Habitat White Myrtle grows in a variety of soils,
including sand, peaty and clayey soils. Its habitats vary
from around watercourses to rocky outcrops and
hillsides (FloraBase, 2016).

Family Myrtaceae.

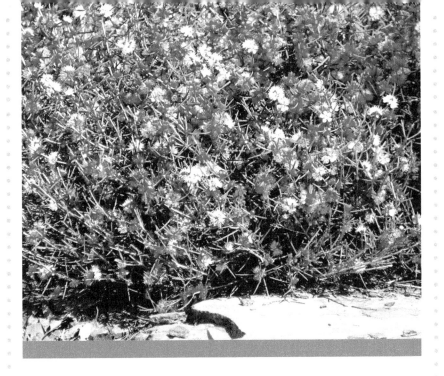

Distribution White Myrtle is found only in the south-west of Western Australia, in coastal and near-coastal areas from the Geraldton Sandplains to Bremer Bay (ANPSA, 2016; FloraBase, 2016).

Parts Used The leaves and twigs.

Medicinal Uses The leaves were crushed and the vapours inhaled to relieve headaches and nasal congestion. The leaves and twigs were crushed and mixed with animal fat and the resulting ointment applied to the skin to treat skin conditions.

Botanical Name *Xylomelum occidentale* R.Br.

Common Name Woody Pear.

Noongar Names Danja, Dumbung, Koongal (Abbott, 1983) and Quabba.

Description Woody Pear grows as a small, twisted shrub or tree 2–8 m in height. It has dark, flaky bark and oak-like leaves. Long, creamy-white, spiky flowers appear in clumps at the end of branchlets from December to February (Birak to early Bunuru). The fruits, as the plant's name suggests, are pear shaped with large woody seeds (FloraBase, 2016; FPCWA, 2016).

Habitat Woody Pear prefers white and grey sand in coastal and near-coastal situations (FloraBase, 2016; FPCWA, 2016).

Distribution Woody Pear is native to Western Australia and is found only in a small area of the south-west, near the coast from Yanchep to Augusta (FloraBase, 2016).

Parts Used The leaves, seeds and bark.

Medicinal Uses Infusions of the leaves and bark were taken internally to relieve pain (Lassak & McCarthy, 2001).

Other Uses The seeds from the fruits were roasted and eaten.

Active Constituents The active constituents are not known for this species, but the wood from some of the genus contains silicic acid (Lassak & McCarthy, 2001).

Family Proteaceae Juss.

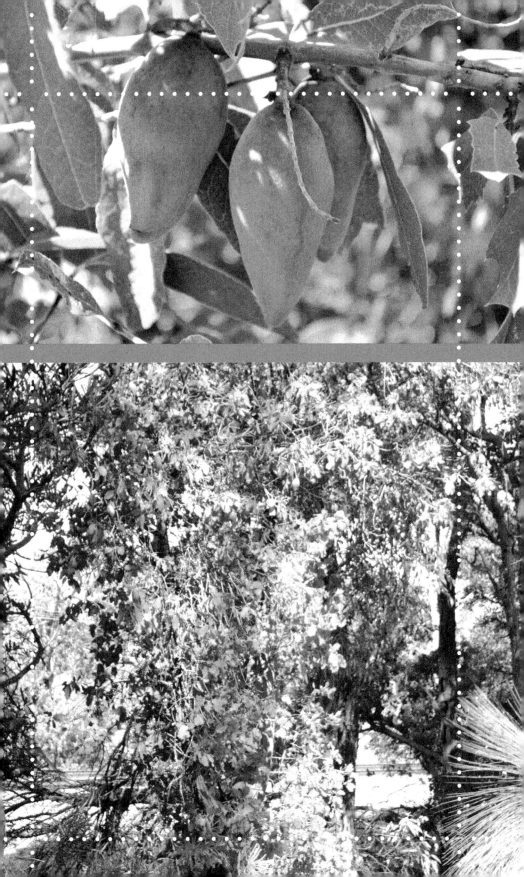

Yanchep Mallee

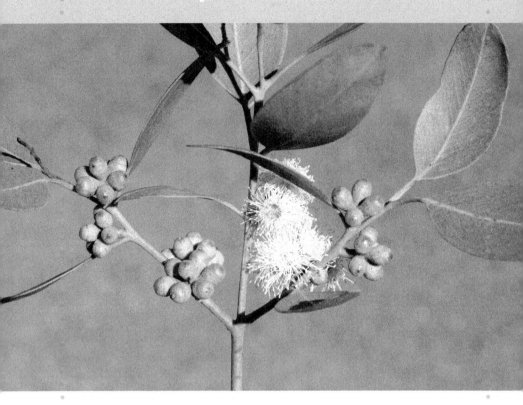

Botanical Name *Eucalyptus argutifolia* Grayling & Brooker.

Common Names Yanchep Mallee and Wabling Hill Mallee.

Noongar Name Moort.

Description Yanchep Mallee is a small Eucalypt that grows only to around 4 m in height. It has smooth, grey to pale copper bark and lance-shaped leaves, which are up to 120 mm long. The white, spiky flowers appear from March to April (late Bunuru to early Djeran). The seed pods are shiny and red to reddish brown (Department of the Environment, 2016; FloraBase, 2016).

Habitat Yanchep Mallee thrives in shallow soils over limestone in coastal and near-coastal situations (Department of the Environment, 2016; FloraBase, 2016).

Family **Myrtaceae Juss.**

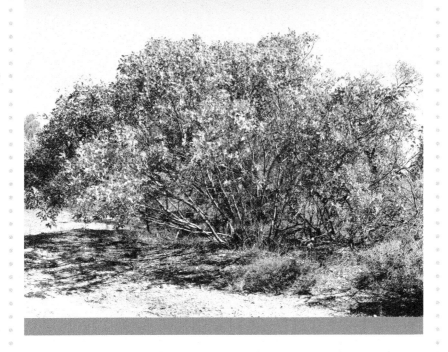

Distribution Yanchep Mallee is native to Western Australia but is becoming rare and endangered due to Perth's urban sprawl. It is known in two locations: on a narrow strip between Wanneroo and Guilderton and at Lake Clifton (Department of the Environment, 2016).

Uses For the Noongar people's use of Eucalypts, see page 24.

Active Constituents For Eucalypts' active constituents, see page 24.

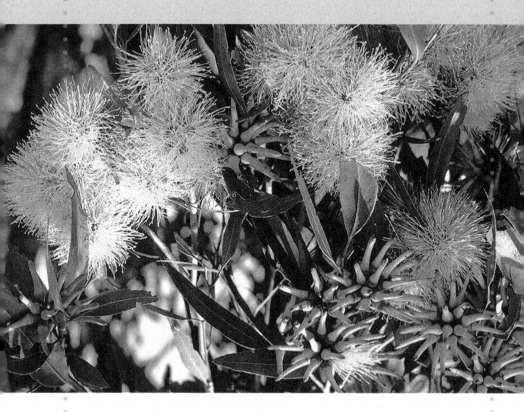

Family Myrtaceae Juss.

Botanical Name *Eucalyptus cornuta* Labill.

Common Name Yate.

Noongar Names Mo, Yandil, Yate and Yeit (Abbott, 1983).

Description Yate is a Eucalypt that grows as a mallee or tree to around 25 m in height. It has rough, dark grey bark on the trunk, with smoother bark on the branches. It produces clusters of long, horn-shaped buds, which are followed by showy clusters of green-yellow flowers from January to May (late Birak to Djeran) or from July to November (late Makuru to Kambarang) (FloraBase, 2016).

Habitat Yate prefers sandy or loamy soils and is found in a variety of habitats including winter-moist areas and rocky outcrops (FloraBase, 2016).

Distribution Yate is native to the south-west of Western

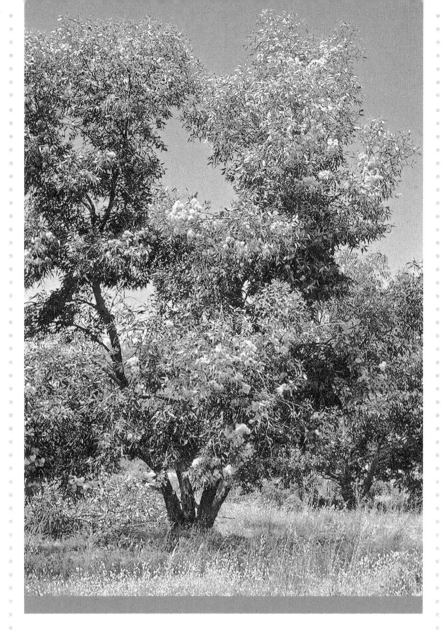

Australia and occurs between Busselton and Albany and around Esperance (FloraBase, 2016).

Parts Used The leaves, gum and bark.

Medicinal Uses Infusions of the bark were drunk to treat diarrhoea. For Eucalypts' other medicinal uses, see page 24.

Active Constituents For Eucalypts' active constituents, see page 24.

York Gum

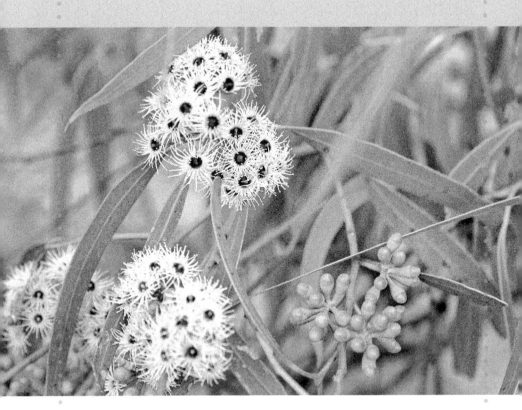

Botanical Name *Eucalyptus loxophleba* Benth.

Common Name York Gum.

Noongar Names Daarwet, Doatta, Goatta, Twotta, Wolung, Yandee (Abbott, 1983 and 1982) and Yorgum.

Description York Gum is a Eucalypt that grows as a mallee to around 5 m or as a tree to 15 m in height. The bark is usually rough and dark grey around the base and smooth and copper coloured further up the tree. The long, lance-shaped leaves are dark green. Small clusters of horn-shaped gumnuts are followed by beautiful clusters of white, spiky flowers from July to December (late Makuru to early Birak) or from January to February (late Birak to early Bunuru) (FloraBase, 2016; FPCWA, 2016).

Habitat York Gum grows in a variety of soils, including sand, clayey, lateritic and dolerite soils. It is found in a variety of

Family **Myrtaceae Juss.**

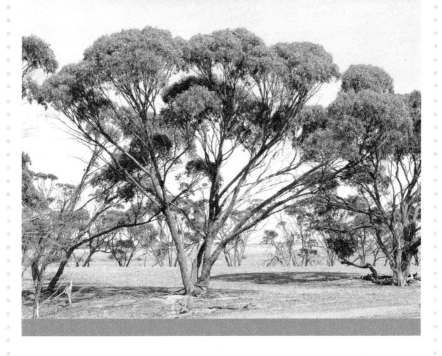

habitats including sandplains, rocky outcrops, on hillsides and around watercourses (FloraBase, 2016).

Distribution York Gum is native to the south-west of Western Australia and has been sighted in coastal and near-coastal areas from Shark Bay to Perth and inland to Albany and Esperance. It is found as far east as Coolgardie. It is very prominent around York – hence the name.

Parts Used The leaves, gum, bark and roots.

Medicinal Uses The gum was crushed to a powder and sprinkled on burns as an antibacterial agent to prevent infection. The leaves were crushed and heated and applied to scorpion stings and insect bites. Roots of the young saplings were pounded into pastes and eaten to relieve upset stomachs. For Eucalypts' other medicinal uses, see page 24.

Other Uses The bark of the roots was used as food in the dry season. The bark was chewed to separate the sweet matter contained in the roots from the leftover residue, which was spat out.

Active Constituents For Eucalypts' active constituents, see page 24.

Appendix Noongar Names for the Identification of Tree Parts

Acacia sap djilyan

Acacia seed kwonart

Acacia tree koonart

Balga tree resin biring

Banksia cone madja

Banksia flower mangatj

Banksia flower species doobarda

Banksia honey djidja

bark boort

berries yurenburt

big leaves doolyaa

Bottlebrush birdak

edible roots or tubers koowin or madja

Eucalyptus glaucous leaf balyoongar

fungus (general term) noomar

green berries mull

gum men or miyan

gum in tree (red) koordan

gum tree ngarnt

gum which is eaten djoolbar

Hakea djanda

medicine bush koorin

roots bwor

small leaves maayal

tree boorn

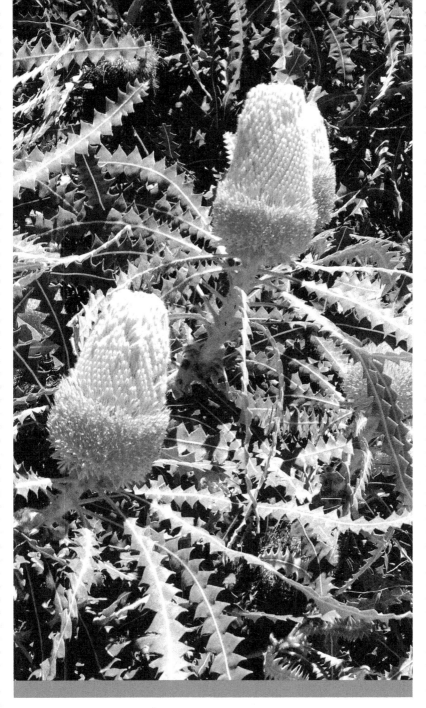

type of flower djet

Wattle tree gum kalyang

Not all of the terms listed below have been used in this book, but for carrying out investigation of traditional herbal medicine it helps to have knowledge of the terms used by herbalists.

anodyne relieves mild pain

anthelmintic a medicine that expels worms

antibilious acts on the bile, relieving biliousness

antiemetic stops vomiting

antiperiodic prevents regular recurrences

antilithic prevents the formation of stones in the urinary organs

antirheumatic relieves or cures rheumatism

antiscorbutic cures or prevents scurvy

antiseptic prevents putrefaction

antispasmodic relieves or prevents spasms

aperient gently laxative without purging

aromatic a stimulant, spicy, anti-griping

astringent causes contraction and arrests discharges

carminative expels wind from the bowels

cathartic evacuates the bowels, a purgative

cholagogue increases the flow of bile into the intestine

decoction a method of extracting dissolved oils, volatile organic compounds and other chemical substances by mashing herbal or plant material, which may include stems, roots, bark and rhizomes, and then boiling them in water

demulcent soothing, relieves inflammation, especially for skin and mucous membranes

deobstruent removes obstruction

depurative purifies the blood

diaphoretic produces perspiration

discutient dissolves and heals tumours

diuretic increases the secretion and flow of urine

emetic produces vomiting

emmenagogue promotes menstruation

emollient softens and soothes inflamed parts when locally applied

esculent edible

expectorant facilitates expulsion of mucus, or phlegm, from the lungs and throat

febrifuge abates and reduces fevers

hepatic pertaining to the liver

infusion a method of extracting desired chemical compounds or flavours from plants by steeping them in a solvent such as water, oil or alcohol

laxative promotes bowel action

lithotriptic dissolves calculi (stones) in the urinary system

nauseant produces vomiting

nervine acts specifically on the nervous system, stops nervous excitement, a tonic

parturient induces and promotes labour at childbirth

pectoral a remedy for chest afflictions

refrigerant cooling

resolvent dissolves boils, tumours and other inflammations

rubefacient increases circulation and produces red skin

sedative quiets nerve action and promotes sleep

steep to soak an item in liquid such as water or alcohol

stomachic excites the action of the stomach, has the effect of strengthening it and relieving indigestion

styptic arrests haemorrhage from cuts

sudorific produces profuse perspiration

tonic a remedy which is invigorating, strengthening and toning

vermifuge expels worms from the intestines

References

Abbott, I. (1983). *Aboriginal Names for Plant Species in South-western Australia*. Technical Paper 5. Perth: Forests Department of Western Australia.

Abbott, T. & Abbott, P. (2015). 'Technical Information'. EucalyptusOil.com. www.eucalyptusoil.com/technical-information.

Ameri, A., Ghadge, C., Vaidya, J. G. & Deokule, S. S. (2011). 'Anti-*Staphylococcus aureus* Activity of *Pisolithus albus* from Pune, India'. *Journal of Medicinal Plants Research*, vol. 5, no. 4, pp. 527–32.

ANBG (Australian National Botanic Gardens). (2002). '*Santalum acuminatum*'. www.anbg.gov.au/gnp/interns-2002/santalum-acuminatum.html.

–– (2013). 'Australian Fungi'. www.anbg.gov.au/fungi/aboriginal.html.

–– (2016a). 'Aboriginal Plant Use Trail'. www.anbg.gov.au/gardens/visiting/exploring/aboriginal-trail/index.html.

–– (2016b). '*Hemigenia incana*'. www.anbg.gov.au/cgi-bin/phtml?p-c=a&pn=20266&size=3.

ANBG & CANBR (Australian National Botanic Gardens & Centre for Australian National Biodiversity Research). (2012). 'Banksias: Genus *Banksia*'. www.cpbr.gov.au/banksia.

ANPSA (Australian Native Plants Society (Australia)) (2016). anpsa.org.au.

Archer, W. (2016). Esperance Wildflowers. esperancewildflowers.blogspot.com.au.

Atlas of Living Australia (2016). bie.ala.org.au.

Australian Native Plants Society (Australia). (2016). Grevillea juncifolia. anpsa.org.au/g-jun.html.

Australian Plants Online (2003). '*Santalum*: A Fascinating Genus'. Australian Native Plants Society (Australia). anpsa.org.au/APOL31/sep03-3.html.

Australian Seed. (2016). www.australianseed.com.

ATRP (Australian Tropical Rainforest Plants). (2010). 6th edn. Australian National Botanic Gardens. www.anbg.gov.au/cpbr/cd-keys/rfk.

BACC (Bunjilaka Aboriginal Cultural Centre). (2016). 'Native Geranium'. Museum Victoria. museumvictoria.com.au/bunjilaka/visiting/milarri-garden/grasses-and-groundcovers/native-geranium.

Beattie, K., Waterman, P. & Leach, D. (2011). '*Centipeda cunninghamii*: An Australian Traditional Medicinal Plant'. Paper presented at the 59th International Congress and Annual Meeting of the Society for Medicinal Plant and Natural Product Research, Antalya, 4–9 September. Abstract published in *Planta Medica*, vol. 77, no. 12, pp. 1379-83.

Bennett, E. (2016). '*Eucalyptus rudis* subsp. *rudis*'. Peppy Plants. www.
    peppyplants.com.au/wp-content/uploads/2012/09/Eucalyptus-rudis.pdf.

Bennett, E. M. (1991). *Common and Aboriginal Names of Western Australian
    Plant Species*. Perth: Wildflower Association of Western Australia.

BGPA (Botanic Gardens & Parks Authority) (2012). 'Plant of the Month:
    November 2012'. [No longer online.]

—— (2015). 'Silver Princess: *Eucalyptus caesia*'. www.bgpa.wa.gov.au/images/
    horticulture/docs/pn_eucalyptus_caesia.pdf.

Bindon, P. (1996). *Useful Bush Plants*. Perth: Western Australian Museum.

Bindon, P. & Chadwick, R. (2011). *A Nyoongar Word List from the South-west
    of Western Australia*. Perth: Western Australian Museum.

BioNET-EAFRINET (2016). Dodonaea viscosa (Sand Olive). keys.lucidcentral.
    org/keys/v3/eafrinet/weeds/key/weeds/Media/Html/Dodonaea_viscosa_
    (Sand_Olive).htm

Bougher, N. (2009). 'Fungi of the Perth Region and Beyond'. Perth Urban
    Bushland Fungi. www.fungiperth.org.au/Download-document/82-Field-
    Book-Part.html.

Bourne, X. (2016). 'Plants of the Denmark Walk Trails: Traditional Noongar
    Names & Uses'. Green Skills. www.greenskills.org.au/pub/pamph/plants.
    html.

Bowman, M., King, D., Reu, S. & Fisher, R. (2000). 'Common Grasses of Central
    Australia'. Land & Water Resources Research & Development Corporation.
    www.southwestnrm.org.au/sites/default/files/uploads/ihub/central-austra-
    lian-grasses.pdf.

BRAIN (Brisbane Rainforest Action and Information Network) (2016). 'Fungi
    Database'. www.brisrain.org.au/01_cms/details.asp?ID=710.

City of Joondalup (2011). 'Plants and People in Mooro Country: Nyungar
    Plant Use in Yellagonga Regional Park'. www.joondalup.wa.gov.au/Files/
    Plants%20and%20People%20in%20Mooro%20Country.pdf.

City of Mandurah (2016). 'Jarrah: *Eucalyptus marginata*'. www.mandurah.
    wa.gov.au/HBItem_186037.PDF.

Collis, R. (2007). Dianella revoluta. www.anbg.gov.au/gnp/interns-2007/dianel-
    la-revoluta.html.

Coppin, P. (2008). 'Nyoongar Food Plant Species'. Peter Coppin. petercoppin.
    com/factsheets/edible/nyoongar.pdf.

Crago, J. (2016). '*Scaevola spinescens* (Maroon Bush, Murin Murin, Prickly Fan
    Flower, Current Bush)'. Bush Medicine. www.bushmedicine.ws/page6.html.

Cribb, A. & Cribb, J. (1983). *Wild Medicine in Australia*. Sydney: Fontana Books.

CSIRO (Commonwealth Scientific and Industrial Research Organisation) (2004). *'Eucalyptus camaldulensis* Dehnh'. Centre for Australian National Biodiversity Research. www.cpbr.gov.au/cpbr/WfHC/Eucalyptus-camaldulensis.

Cunningham, I. (1998). *The Trees That Were Nature's Gift*. Perth: Environmental Printing Company.

–– (2005). *The Land of Flowers: An Australian Environment on the Brink*. Brighton Le Sands: Otford Press.

Customary Medicinal Knowledgebase (2011). Publisher/host. [No longer online.] (was Macquarie Universit the link was www.biolinfo.org/cmkb/)

Daw, B., Walley, T. & Keighery, G. (2011). *Bush Tucker Plants of the South-West*. Kensington: Department of Environment and Conservation.

Department of Primary Industry (WA) (2010). 'Old Man Saltbush'. www.dpi.nsw.gov.au/agriculture/resources/private-forestry/paddock-plants/Atriplex-nummularia-Old-Man-Saltbush.pdf.

Department of the Environment (Australia) (2016). *'Eucalyptus argutifolia*: Yanchep Mallee, Wabling Hill Mallee'. www.environment.gov.au/cgi-bin/sprat/public/publicspecies.pl?taxon_id=24263.

eFloraSA (Electronic Flora of South Australia) (2013). www.flora.sa.gov.au/factsheets.html.

EKSA (Environmental Knowledge Systems Australia) (n.d.). 'Soapbush'. [No longer online.] (last seen working 2015)

EucaLink (2004). PlantNET. plantnet.rbgsyd.nsw.gov.au/PlantNet/Euc/index.html.

Feng, Y., Wang, N., Zhu, M., Feng, Y., Li, H. & Tsao, S. (2011). 'Recent Progress on Anticancer Candidates in Patents of Herbal Medicinal Products'. *Recent Patents on Food, Nutrition & Agriculture*, vol. 3, no. 1, pp. 30–48.

Flora of Australia Online. (2016). Australian National Botanic Gardens. www.anbg.gov.au/abrs/online-resources/flora.

Florabank. (2016). www.florabank.org.au.

FloraBase. (2016). florabase.dec.wa.gov.au.

FPCWA (Forest Products Commission Western Australia). (2016). www.fpc.wa.gov.au.

FQPB (Friends of the Queens Park Bushland). (2011). *'Xanthorrhoea preissii'*. www.friendsofqueensparkbushland.org.au/xanthorrhoea-preissii.

Frawley, W. (2004). *International Encyclopedia of Linguistics*. 2nd edn. Melbourne: Oxford University Press.

French, M. (2012). *Eucalypts of Western Australia's Wheatbelt*. Perth: Malcolm French.

Gardening Australia (2011). 'Fact Sheet: *Xanthorrea*'. ABC. www.abc.net.au/gardening/stories/s1145455.htm.

Glasby, M. (2015). 'Aboriginal Medicine'. Western Australia Now and Then. www.wanowandthen.com/Aboriginal-Medicine.html.

Greening Australia (2016). '*Geranium solanderi*'. www.greeningaustralia.org.au/uploads/knowledge-portal/Geranium_solanderi.pdf.

Grice, I., Rogers, K. & Griffiths, L. (2011). 'Isolation of Bioactive Compounds that Relate to the Anti-platelet Activity of *Cymbopogon ambiguous*'. *Evidence-based Complementary and Alternative Medicine*, vol. 2011, article 467134, www.hindawi.com/journals/ecam.

HerbiGuide (2014). 'Common Bracken'. www.herbiguide.com.au/Descriptions/hg_Common_Bracken.htm.

HLPG (Hills Local Permaculture Group) (2010). 'Aboriginal Bush Medicine'. PermacultureWest. permaculturewest.org.au/community/local-groups/hlpg/hlpg_july_2010_newsletter.pdf.

Isaacs, J. (2009). *Bush Food: Aboriginal Food and Herbal Medicine*. Sydney: New Holland.

Knott, L. (2012). 'Cachexia'. Patient. patient.info/doctor/cachexia.

Lassak, E. & McCarthy, T. (2001). *Australian Medicinal Plants*. Sydney: New Holland.

Leithhead, B. (2016). 'Fungi Photos Group P: *Phlebopus marginatus* to *Podoscypha petalodes*'. Bill Leithhead. www.elfram.com/fungi/fungipics_p.html.

Monash University (2010). 'Aboriginal Plants in the Grounds of Monash University'. [No longer online.]

Natural Cancer Treatment (2015). '*Scaevola spinescens*: A Traditional Bush Medicine'. naturalcancertreatment.org/about.

NBLC (Noongar Boodjar Language Centre) (2014). 'Noongar Dialects'. noongarboodjar.com.au/language/noongar-dialects.

NMNR (Nyalar Mirungan-ah Nature Refuge) (2013). 'Plants Used By Aboriginal People'. Cicada Woman Tours. cicadawoman.weebly.com/uploads/8/7/3/4/8734418/plants_used_by_aboriginal_people_april_2013.pdf.

NQ Dry Tropics (2015). 'Dodder Laurel'. wiki.bdtnrm.org.au/index.php/Dodder_Laurel.

NSWFO (New South Wales Flora Online) (2016). PlantNET. plantnet.rbgsyd.nsw. gov.au.

Olive Pink Botanic Garden. (2010). Medicinal and Bush Food Plants. opbg.com. au/wp-content/uploads/2010/03/Medicinal-and-Bushfood-plants.pdf.

Oz Native Plants (2016). www.oznativeplants.com.

Pearn, J. (2004). 'Medical Ethnobotany of Australia: Past and Present'. Paper presented to the Linnean Society, London, 30 September. Transcript published by University of Queensland. espace.library.uq.edu.au/eserv. php?pid=UQ:10307&dsID=jp_meia_ls_04.pdf.

Peile, A. (1997). *Body and Soul: An Aboriginal View*. Perth: Hesperian Press.

Perth Seed (2010). www.perthseed.com.

Plant Broome (2016). '*Solanum lasiophyllum*'. www.plantbroome.com.au/ plant_detail.php?plant_id=148.

Rainbow Coast (2015). 'South Coast Seasons Calendar'. www.rainbowcoast. com.au/areas/rainbowcoast/seasons.htm.

Readford, H. (2011). '*Pisolithus* sp.' BushcraftOz. bushcraftoz.com/forums/ showthread.php?7264-Pisolithus-sp&s=d2b0b887fc7c3de0cf9befa595d 28fb3.

Rippey, E. & Rowland, B. (1995). *Plants of the Perth Coast and Islands.* Perth: University of Western Australia Press.

Robinson, R. (2007). '*Pisolithus albus*: White Dye-ball'. Fungus Fact Sheet 9. Department of Environment and Conservation (WA). Published by Department of Parks and Wildlife (WA). www.dpaw.wa.gov.au/images/ documents/about/science/fungus/9_2007-03_Pisolithus_albus_DEC_FF.pdf.

Royal Botanic Gardens & Domain Trust (n.d.). *Cymbopogon obtectus.* www. rbgsyd.nsw.gov.au/education/Resources/bush_foods/Cymbopogon_ obtectus. (Webpage no longer available. Last year seen working was 2015)

Royal Botanic Gardens & Domain Trust (n.d.). *Pteridium esculentum.* www.rbgsyd. nsw.gov.au/education/Resources/bush_foods/Pteridium_esculentum. (Webpage no longer available. Last year seen working was 2015)

Saj, P. & Thoppil, J. (2011). 'Chemical Composition and Antimicrobial Properties of Essential Oil of Agonis Flexuosa'. *International Journal of Institutional Pharmacy and Life Sciences*, vol. 1, no. 2, pp. 12–17. www.ijipls.com/ uploaded/journal_files/110907110955.pdf.

SERCUL (South East Regional Centre for Urban Landcare) (2014a). 'Bush Tucker Plants for Your Home Garden'. www.sercul.org.au/bushtucker/BushTucker-Brochure2014.pdf.

—— (2014b). 'Traditional Bush Tucker Plant Fact Sheets'. www.sercul.org.au/bushtucker/BushTuckerPlantFactSheets.pdf.

Survival.org.au (2011). *'Typha'*. www.survival.org.au/bf_typha.php.

Taste Australia (2016). 'Bush Remedies'. tasteaustralia.biz/bushfood/bush-remedies.

Tindale, N. (1940). *Map Showing the Distribution of the Aboriginal Tribes of Australia*. Adelaide: Government Photolithographer.

TSU (Threatened Species Unit, Department of Primary Industries, Water and Environment (Tas.)) (2016). *'Centipeda cunninghamii'*. Department of Primary Industries, Parks, Water and Environment (Tas.). www.dpipwe.tas.gov.au/inter.nsf/Attachments/SSKA-72Y8F7/$FILE/Centipeda%20cunninghamii.pdf.

UniServe Science (2012). 'Aboriginal Use of Native Plants: Marri'. science.uniserve.edu.au/school/curric/stage4_5/nativeplants/gallery/marri/index.html.

Venkatesh, S., Reddy, Y., Ramesh, M., Swamy, M., Mahadevan, N. & Suresh, B. (2008). 'Pharmacognostical Studies on *Dodonaea viscosa* Leaves'. *African Journal of Pharmacy and Pharmacology*, vol. 2, no. 4, pp. 83–8.

Wikipedia (2015). *'Eucalyptus cornuta'*. en.wikipedia.org/wiki/Eucalyptus_cornuta.

WNRM (Wheatbelt Natural Resource Management) (2009). *'Nyungar Budjara Wangany*: Nyungar NRM Wordlist and Language Collection Booklet of the Avon Catchment Region'. www.wheatbeltnrm.org.au/sites/default/files/knowledge_hub/documents/nyungar-dictionary.pdf.

World Wide Wattle (2013). 'Wattle Uses'. www.worldwidewattle.com/schools/uses.php.

—— (2016). worldwidewattle.com/speciesgallery/browse.php?l=a.

YMNAI (Yelakitj Moort Nyungar Association Incorporated) (2008). 'Bushtucker/Medicine'. home.iprimus.com.au/hecatej/yelakitj/bushtucker.html.